It's A Matter of Life and Death:

Growing Up in a Funeral Home and What I Learned Since

No one clamors to read about death and funerals, but people have a curiosity about what happens in funeral homes – even though they don't necessarily want to live in one. A frequent question I got as a boy was, 'How can you live there?' It was easy. My sister Marianne and I never knew anything different than living over one. It was a blessing though. It taught us about life and about what truly matters – finding happiness and peace.

"This is not a puff piece. *It's a Matter of Life and Death* is comprehensive and could easily be part of a reference series every family should have. It is an extensive treatment of the subject I have not seen in any other publication."

— **EDWARD F. POOLE MD, FACS**

It's A Matter of Life and Death:

Growing Up in a Funeral Home and What I Learned Since

LAWRENCE J. DANKS

Dedicated to the Cast of Characters:
My Father, My Mother, My Sister Marianne
and Jack Marinella

Author's Note

My father sold his funeral home in the mid-1970s. It has been in continuous operation since then and is now operated by a funeral director our family has high regard for. My sister and I chose the current owner to conduct the funerals for our parents.

Neither my sister nor I have had any connection with the business since my father's retirement. Anything I relate here is solely based on my experience there prior to then.

My purpose in writing the book is to provide insight into funerals and what it was like living in a funeral home. More importantly, it offers suggestions to make going through both life and death experiences more beneficial.

Table of Contents

PART I

Seeking Happiness

Nobody Gets Out Alive:
It's Important to Live Well in the Meantime

WE'RE ALL DYING FROM THE DAY WE GET HERE. A SHORT TIME BEFORE his impending death, writer William Saroyan had a different hope:

"Everybody has to die. I always believed an exception would be made in my case. Now what?"

There probably are many things we can't agree on, but whether we're going to die or not isn't one of them. The focus should never be on dying though. It should be on living and optimizing whatever time we have left.

As far as an afterlife goes, I'm comfortable believing what I believe, just like most of you probably are – whatever your beliefs. I believe that there's more, and that after we die, we're headed to an eternal home. It's good to have something to aspire to. When viewed as a renewed opportunity to be reunited with those we care about, it offers some additional comfort. We shouldn't be in any hurry though. We're meant to enjoy this world, and to try not to hurt anybody along the way.

To some I know this seems silly, but it works for me, especially when I've lost loved ones and friends. It provides the hope that their loss will only be temporary. Even for those who don't believe in an afterlife, anyone should find the reasoning of the great mathematician Blaise Pascal something to ponder. He said we lose nothing by believing – even if we find later that there is nothing after death – but nothingness. On the other hand, if we don't believe and there is something there, we might wish we had.

Some Differing Points of View

IN AN ENGAGING PBS SPECIAL, "INTO THE NIGHT: PORTRAITS OF LIFE and Death," there are segments in which individuals express their opinions about death.

In "The Mortician," Caitlan Doughty (Alternative Mortician), who had the uncommon insight of working in a crematorium, joined a movement to make death more visible by going to "death salons" and "death cafes" in Switzerland and England. One clip showed her speaking to an audience that seemed much more lighthearted than you might imagine. She thought we needed to gain more understanding of death. She described her own death saying, "I sail off into nothingness – like the end of a film reel going white and flapping." While not a religious believer, she said, "We need ritual around death." Then she cited how cultures around the world have varied ones to help remove some of the pain from it.

In another segment, "The Storyteller," Jim Crace, a writer, felt a great loss from the death of his father. He said, "I wish I was religious." While he said religion has some chinks in it, it does provide some armor to protect us from the pain of death. He said it was important to find some real comfort, even if it's partially fictional. That's very true. Losing a loved one is too traumatic to go it alone. Spiritual support, or even fictional or mental constructs, can be very helpful.

Mr. Crace said his father wanted no funeral, flowers, or anything else. Afterward, he found an acorn in his father's coat pocket. It reminded him of the many others he used to carry, which he dropped along the way when he took walks with him. He crushed them underfoot, so they would grow into the giant oaks in Britain that last for four to five hundred years. He said we can't deal with death in its entirety, but he was consoled that, in continuity, there was a future. Regardless of your own belief, we may similarly find things to console us if we look for them.

More about funerals and funeral homes later. That can teach us a lot about life. Life, obviously, isn't just about death though, so let's look at how we can make a better life for ourselves.

The Search for Happiness

ONE THING WE CAN AGREE ON IS THAT WE WANT TO BE HAPPY WHILE we're here. It doesn't mean that we'll be smiling all the time. The realism of living daily life presents circumstances that make that virtually impossible. So are we on our own with how to find happiness?

Fortunately, there's a large and growing body of knowledge from positive psychology that provides us with the elements we should seek to find a good and happy life – and also to learn what is not likely to produce it over the long term.

Positive psychology is the relatively recent creation of a number of noted psychologists, principal among them, Dr. Martin Seligman, author of *Authentic Happiness,* and subsequently, *Flourish.* He felt that psychology needed to go beyond simply dealing with problems of depression and mental illness, and move toward a new and more positive study of what's most likely to produce well-being in our lives. I'd recommend reading both books, in order. They provide excellent guides for living.

The wonderful thing about the research positive psychologists have done is now people don't have to slog along in the dark trying to find their way to happiness and well-being. Recognized, research-based principles are available to facilitate the journey. Sometimes they run counter to what we might think.

Seligman says, *"When well-being comes from engaging in our strengths and virtues, our lives are imbued with authenticity. [...]* When you read about strengths, you will find some that are deeply characteristic of you, whereas others are not. I call the former your *'signature strengths',* and one of my purposes is to distinguish these strengths from those that are less a part of you. I do not believe that you should devote overly much effort to correcting your weaknesses. Rather, I believe that the highest success in living, and the deepest emotional satisfaction, comes from building and using your signature strengths." (As the famed financier and adviser to presidents Bernard Baruch said, "Do what you do best and leave the rest to others.") "The ability to attach yourself to something larger, and the larger the entity to which you attach yourself the better, the more meaning you will add to your life." (A common thread I've found in many self-help books.)

Such meaning boils down to serving the needs of others, rather than serving yourself or doing things that are ego-driven. This can make a great contribution to your happiness and feeling of success in life. And you don't have to be someone professionally dedicated to serving the spiritual needs of others or a social worker to do this. Anyone can do it in small ways in daily life. Effectively, when we help others, we help ourselves.

Mother Teresa attached herself to something larger than she was. She was asked how she could do the work she and her sisters did, bringing the sick and dying into their hospital from the streets of Kolkata, so they could be bathed, treated, and die with dignity. Many of those who were brought in had lived on the streets their whole lives and had never slept in a bed. She replied that if she were doing this for herself, she could not have done it for very long. It was only possible because she was "doing it for Christ," – the higher purpose that was important to her. You don't have to do something higher for religious or spiritual reasons, although you may, only for a higher reason that is meaningful to you.

The kindnesses don't have to be large. My mother used to say, "Everyone wants to do the big things, but no one wants to do the little things." She told me a story she heard about a young boy walking along the beach seeing hundreds of starfish that had washed up and gotten stranded there when the tide went out. The boy starting picking them up and, one by one, threw them back into the ocean. A man came along and saw him doing it and said, "There are hundreds of these things here. What possible difference can you hope to make?" The boy picked another one up and threw it back and said, "It makes a difference to this one." That was Mother Teresa's philosophy – one, one, one. Do what you can do.

Don't worry about the whole. Just do your part. This was the first story I told when I gave my mother's eulogy. It was the way she lived her life.

Authentic Happiness:
Identifying Your Signature Strengths

IDENTIFY YOUR SIGNATURE STRENGTHS. *GO TO THE AUTHENTIC HAPPINESS* website at the University of Pennsylvania: www.authentichappiness .sas.upenn.edu.

Click on "Questionnaires" at the top. In the middle column, you will see the "VIA Survey of Character Strengths." It surveys twenty-four possible character strengths. After you finish the test, you'll know what your signature strengths are. I've taken the test twice. It described me well.

Authentic Happiness contains interpretive information that provides further guidance. Your signature strengths are the ones you should try to use as much as possible in your daily life, including when you're at work.

If you're an employer or manager, choose candidates whose signature strengths match the work they do and make room to allow employees to re-craft their work, within the bounds of your organizational objectives.

Do you remember the children's Fisher-Price Workbench, where a child took a small hammer and pounded square, rectangular, and round pegs into the appropriate holes? What happened when kids tried to bang the square peg into the round hole? It created a non-productive and frustrating situation. It's the same with people on the job. Put square pegs into square holes and round pegs into round holes as much as possible. You won't have to pound the life out of them. They'll fit right in. Increased productivity and employee well-being can be the result.

No one else on earth, out of billions of people, has the same combination of signature strengths, in the same proportions you have. *These unique talents are too beautiful and meaningful to waste. Your potential happiness is too beautiful to waste, too.* When you are living your best life, it benefits you and anyone who comes into contact with you.

Lasting Happiness

DR. SELIGMAN SAYS, *"IT IS IMPORTANT TO DISTINGUISH MOMENTARY happiness from your enduring level of happiness."* There is a difference between something pleasurable and something that provides true gratification. While eating ice cream sundaes every day or making more money might produce happiness, they are not the source of long-term happiness produced by gratification-producing experiences.

"Habitually choosing the easy pleasures over the gratifications may have untoward consequences. One of the major symptoms of depression is self-absorption." This is fairly observable when we see high-profile examples of some athletes and celebrities, who often spend millions of dollars and have the freedom to do just about anything they want, having drug, alcohol, and behavioral problems.

Positive psychologists aren't saying that pleasure isn't a good thing to have in your life, but focusing on it alone will not make you happy. Pleasure is transitory. Gratification produces real and substantive support for finding long-term happiness.

The Importance of Resilience

INTO EVERY LIFE, A LITTLE RAIN, AND SOMETIMES A LOT OF IT, WILL FALL. *No matter what you are subject to, no matter how bad it is right now, or later in life, it didn't come to stay, it came to pass.* Psychological research is on your side. Recovery often occurs within a few months. Just keep moving forward. Whenever you get low, remember the famous song lyrics, "Time Is on Your Side, Oh Yes It Is." In my "Principles of Management" lecture course, I accompany this with a "slip-sliding" dance, not to be simple, but to reinforce the important message to always keep hope alive – no matter what happens in your life.

People can be remarkably resilient. Not long before finishing this book, I met two amazing women at a St. Patrick's Day Irish Breakfast. The first woman lost her son in a car accident. The other woman had a terminal kidney disease and required a transplant. She had been on the transplant list for over four years. She became the recipient of the young man's kidneys. She and the boy's mother have become fast friends. She even travels with their family.

Many received his other organs, including a woman who received his heart. She has had three children since, children she never could have had without the transplant. Out of tragedy, sometimes good things can come.

Moving Ahead

PASSION AND PERSEVERANCE IS WHAT ACCORDING TO PENN PSYCHOLOGY Professor, Dr. Angela Duckworth, creates *Grit*, the title of her fascinating book. Being "grittier" (persevering to achieve a meaningful goal) can be a strong determinant in achieving success. She says, "You can grow your own grit from the inside out: You can cultivate your interests. You can develop a daily challenge-exceeding skill practice. You can connect your work to a purpose beyond yourself. And you can learn to hope when all seems lost."

You can also grow your grit "from the outside in. Parents, coaches, teachers, bosses, mentors, friends – developing your personal grit depends critically on other people."

Another book that can be helpful in making changes and getting yourself on an improved path is the best seller, *The Power of Habit* by Charles Duhigg. Many times, the ruts we find ourselves in are a result of non-productive habits we want to change. Duhigg explains the process and shows how to replace bad habits with good ones.

You'll frequently find that the solution to improving your life is in your hands. But sometimes we get in our own way. As Pogo, the famous comic strip character said, "We have met the enemy, and he is us."

Similarly Ben Stein, the economist and comedian said, "Most of the problems we have are right between our ears." Psychologists can help us with those when we need it. There is no shame in asking for help with re-framing and clarifying our situation. The shame is in needing help and not asking for it.

Don't dwell on negative things. Move along and move ahead. *When a negative thought keeps entering your head, just say to yourself, "No! Don't go there!" And distract yourself as often as you need to by doing something positive.*

Sometimes inertia can be caused by things that are emotionally paralyzing. My mother counseled many people during her lifetime. Her advice when someone couldn't seem to move forward: "Just do the next thing." Don't mentally overwhelm yourself. So if you feel as if you can hardly move, get your shower. Then take care of your personal grooming. Then unload the dishwasher. *Don't think of everything, just think of one thing – the next thing.* Keep moving down the track – one item at a time. This can serve to distract you from your funk. After a while, you will sense some degree of progress, to the point where you may be able to start seeing some light at the end of the tunnel. Keep moving toward it – even if you have to crawl sometimes.

The Importance of Gratitude

HAVING GRATITUDE MAKES IT EASIER TO ABSORB THE SHOCKS OF LIFE. Focus on a higher calling and have gratitude – the dynamic duo for finding more satisfaction in life. Knowing it and doing it aren't the same. It's something we all need to work on.

Flow and Gratification

FLOW IS A BOOK BY THE RECOGNIZED FATHER OF THE CONCEPT, MIHALY Czikszentmihalyi. Being in a "flow state" means doing something meaningful and challenging that has clear goals, when we lose the concept of time and self. Increasing the frequency of "flow states" increases gratification, and that increases well-being.

Flourish: A Visionary New Understanding of Happiness and Well-Being

THROUGH FURTHER INVESTIGATION, RESEARCH AND CONSIDERATION, Dr. Seligman says in *Flourish* that "happiness underexplains what we choose [...] that the modern ear immediately hears "happy" to mean buoyant mood, merriment, good cheer and smiling." He says, "The gold standard for measuring well-being is flourishing, and that the goal of positive psychology is to increase flourishing," not happiness alone, although he includes happiness in his theory of well-being.

Seligman's well-being theory has five elements (PERMA):

POSITIVE EMOTION: "Happiness and life satisfaction [...] are now demoted from being the goal of the entire theory, to being one of the factors included under the element of positive emotion."

ENGAGEMENT + Flow

POSITIVE RELATIONSHIPS: When asked what, in two words or fewer, positive psychology is about, Christopher Peterson, a University of Michigan psychology professor and one of the founders of positive psychology replied, "Other people. Other people are the best antidote to the downs of life and the single most reliable up." Seligman says, "We scientists have found that doing a kindness produces the single most reliable momentary increase in well-being of any exercise we tested." Aldous Huxley said the same thing: "People often asked me what is the most effective technique for transforming their life. It is a little embarrassing, that after years and years of research and experimentation, I have to say that the best answer is – just be a little kinder." My kindness book, *Your*

Unfinished Life: The Classic and Timeless Guide to Finding Happiness and Success Through Kindness is contained in one of the latter sections of my *Happiness, Well-Being and Success* website mentioned below.

MEANING: Belonging to and serving something larger than the self.

ACCOMPLISHMENT (Achievement): "Is often pursued for its own sake, even when it brings no positive emotion, no meaning, and nothing in the way of positive relationships."

More details and supporting information are contained in the books mentioned above. What I've presented here, combined with my website below and the list of recommended resources at the end of this book will lead you to many other excellent self-help sources. It's more than enough to get you going on your own road to improved well-being.

Happiness, Well-Being and Success Website

MY WEBSITE IS DEVOTED TO FINDING HAPPINESS, WELL-BEING AND success, as well as offering suggestions for innovation, motivation and reinvention. It contains summaries of many books and articles, as well as some of my own. I hope it will help you, your family and friends in your lives. Log into the website through Camden County College, the institution where I currently teach:

Log into: ccc.webstudy.com
Click the "X" in the "How To Login" box
User Name: happiness
Password: success
Click on Happiness, Motivation and Success, then "Timeline" and then "Expand All"

The purpose of the website is to provide a bridge to fuller exposure to positive psychology and other self-help reading. It is not just for college students. It's for anyone seeking more out of life. (Any subsequent changes to the website's location will be indicated on my LinkedIn Page: Lawrence J. Danks.)

Plan to Live to Be One Hundred

THE WELL-KNOWN MOTIVATIONAL SPEAKER AND EVANGELIST DR. Robert Schuller said, "We should plan to live to be one hundred." This might sound like a long overreach because most people don't get to be centenarians. That's not what it really means though. What it does mean is that *we should consistently have goals to strive for*. A Japanese proverb confirms this, "Only staying active will make you want to live a hundred years."

Jack was a friend of my father's who lived to be one hundred and three. People always called my father "Mr. Danks" or "Tom", but his far older friend called him "Tommy". Even in his seventies, to him my father was a "mere youth", as my stepmother Helen used to say about me when I was in my fifties.

I don't think Jack thought much about how long he would live. He had a mustache and chain-smoked hefty cigars. He always wore flannel shirts with the pocket stuffed with about five or six of them. If he ever heard warnings about smoking and longevity, he didn't pay any attention to them. He just stayed active running his business in Philadelphia until the closing years of his life. He always walked with purpose and was never short of opinions. Staying engaged, a good step and a sharp mind. They were habits he had that are good to emulate.

I spoke with my mother about her situation when she was in the hospital for six weeks before she died. I asked her, "What do you think about all this?" She simply said that she trusted in God and was just going to follow along with whatever happened. The main thing is to come to peace with life and to set a good example while you're doing it. My mother's attitude has served as a model for me. I'm much less concerned about dying than I might have been otherwise. It's easier to be philosophical about all this when you're not facing your own earthly end, so I'll have to wait and see how I do.

How will you know when *your work* is done? The answer is *you're never done as long as you're still breathing.* My mother was still "doing good", even in her final hours. I learned that her substantially younger roommate told her about some concerns she was having. She said later how helpful my mother's advice had been. So we can even "do good" from our deathbed. The night my mother was dying, the hospital staff offered to move her roommate out of the room, but she said that she wanted to stay with my mother. What a thoughtful way to return the good that was shown to her.

You Probably Have a Lot of Time Left

ONE OF MY FAVORITE WRITERS IS TOM BUTLER-BOWDON. TOM IS A master at summarizing classic works in his series "50 Classics" – books on self-help, psychology, success, business, economics, politics, prosperity, and philosophy. I recommend all of them as tremendous tools for education, self-development, and motivation. They are well written and can help us catch up on many books we would have liked to read, or should have read, but didn't.

In a non-series book, *Never Too Late to Be Great: The Power of Thinking Long*, Tom makes the words, "There's no sense trying. I'll never make it," or "I'm too old for that," obsolete. No one could ever believe that about themselves after reading all the inspirational stories in his book. *No one is exempt from outside events, but most of us have more time than we might imagine.*

Never Too Late to Be Great rests on two simple observations:

– All great accomplishments may take longer than we first imagined.

– It's rarely too late to begin something great. A woman in the Philadelphia area started painting at seventy and was having an exhibition of her work when she was a hundred. How cool is that? "Increasing longevity should make us think again. You realize that, '*Yes, I do have more time.*'" *But don't push it and don't pressure yourself and cause stress.* That could give you less time!

We often hear about people getting "second chances" in life but "the good news is that across a longish lifespan, most of us are not just given a second chance, but possibly a third or even a fourth chance to succeed at what we really want to do." Encouraging, isn't it?

Sixty Minutes reported that ninety-year-olds are the fastest growing population group percentage-wise today. Act as if you could be one of them. Make plans for whatever is important to you and take whatever steps are necessary to make it happen.

Age can sometimes be a limiter. At seventy-three, I'm not going to be a physician or a wide receiver now, but there are still some possibilities open to me. There certainly are far more available to you.

John, a high school classmate in the class after me, died of a heart attack while paddle boarding – still living life to the end. He was a good model for "it's never too late." He was a starter on our Gloucester Catholic 1964 NJ State Championship basketball team and received a full scholarship to a well-known Eastern university, where he majored in accounting. He went on to work for a "Big Eight" accounting firm for a few years, then decided that he wanted to be an orthopedic surgeon. He effectively started over, leaving a successful career with good prospects behind and went on to create an orthopedic practice in Southern California that lasted until his untimely passing. Decisions like this take forethought but don't think that it's not possible. The younger you are, the more options you have. It may take time, and it will take patience.

Have a Purpose

IN *IKIGAI: THE JAPANESE SECRET TO A LONG AND HAPPY LIFE*, THE authors Hector Garcia and Francesc Miralles define "ikigai" as "the reason we get up in the morning." They provide lessons from centenarians, identifying many things that lead to a long and happy life. They conducted one hundred interviews with the eldest members of a village in Okinawa, an island that has the highest percentage of older people in the world. Here's some of their advice about what's important:

Don't worry. "Smile, open your heart to people." Avoid anxiety and stress.

Cultivate good habits. "Working. If you don't work, your body breaks down."

Nurture your friendships every day. "Talk each day with the people you love. That's the secret to a long life."

Live an unhurried life. "Slow down" and "Relax." "You live much longer if you are not in a hurry." "Do many different things every day. Always stay busy, but do one thing at a time without getting overwhelmed." (In spite of what many think, research has shown that "multi-tasking" is not effective.) "The secret to a long life is going to bed early and getting up early, and going for a walk. Living peacefully and enjoying the little things."

Be optimistic. "I'm ninety-eight, but consider myself young. I still have so much to do." "Laugh. Laughter is the most important thing. I laugh wherever I go."

Ikigai contains many anti-aging secrets, tells how to find flow in everything you do, and offers suggestions for diet, healthful exercises, and avoiding stress and worry. It's an excellent guide.

Take Care of Your Head

WHILE IT MAY BE TRITE TO SAY THAT "YOU ARE WHAT YOU THINK," IT'S become an axiom because of the obvious truth in it. Dr. Catherine Sanderson, Manwell Family Professor in Life Sciences (Psychology) at Amherst College, who was featured on a segment of *Sixty Minutes,* says in her book, *The Positive Shift: Mastering Mindset to Improve Happiness, Health and Longevity:* "The truth is, the way we think about ourselves and the world around us dramatically impacts our happiness, health, how fast or slow we age, and even how long we live. In fact, people with a positive mindset about aging live on average 7.5 years longer than those without." (That's a big bump, so maybe it's time to revisit some of our traditional thinking.)

"That might sound alarming to those of us who struggle to see the bright side, but the good news is we can make surprisingly simple changes or small shifts to how we think, feel, and act that will really pay off. " Sanderson shows how our mindset—or thought pattern—exerts a substantial influence on our psychological and physical health[...]no matter what our natural tendency, with practice we can make minor tweaks in our mindset that will improve the quality—and longevity—of our life.

The Positive Shift gives readers practical and easy strategies for changing maladaptive thought patterns and behaviors so they can live longer, happier lives. These behaviors include: appreciating nature, giving to others and spending money on experiences and not possessions – an excellent justification for my traveling more and living with my older automobile ☺. Sanderson says, "Living your best life is truly mind over matter. Believe in yourself and rethink your way to a happier reality."

Take Care of Your Health

IT'S IMPORTANT TO TAKE CARE OF YOUR HEALTH. SEE YOUR DOCTOR several times a year, get recommended screenings and blood tests, get proper rest and nutrition, and find productive ways to deal with stress.

I've heard of people who don't want to get mammograms or co-lonoscopies because they're "afraid they might find something" or that "they're uncomfortable." Dying from cancer hurts a lot more. To say nothing of a life cut short. Sometimes things happen to us we have no control over, but at least we should take the offensive against what we have some ability to influence.

Health issues are like basements. If left unattended too long, they get to a point where we can't keep up with it all. Deal with health matters promptly when they arise. Get ahead and stay ahead.

On Exercise

FROM ABC'S *GOOD MORNING AMERICA*, REPORTED BY DR. JOHN BYUN of *ABC's Medical Unit:*

Even short bursts of exercise can reduce Americans' risk of disease and death says a study by researchers at the National Cancer Institute and the National Institutes of Health. "Virtually all [studies] report that higher volume of moderate or vigorous physical activity, whether performed intermittently or in sustained bouts, lowers all-cause mortality," wrote Deborah Rohm Young and William L. Haskell in an editorial accompanying research published in the *Journal of the American Heart Association*.

The new study finds that the length of each episode of exercise is unrelated to the benefit seen in living longer. Researchers said that a mere five minutes of jogging counts toward better health.

Getting about sixty minutes per day of moderate to vigorous physical activity *cuts the risk of death over the time period by half. Getting about 100 minutes per day cuts the risk to approximately 75 percent* – and it is the total time moving, not the length of exercise that matters.

It appears that protecting our life span may be easier than we thought. I wish I could tell you that I exercise. I don't. I do walk up to the third floor to get to my office and take occasional walks. I save my real walks for miles in France. I walked eighty-five miles in about twenty days on my recent trip there. In all seriousness, if you already do these good things, keep doing them. If you don't, start. It can get you closer to living until you're one hundred!

Better Sleep and Better Habits Can Help

HOW OFTEN HAVE YOU HEARD OTHERS SAY THEY'RE TIRED? HOW often do you feel that way? One of the keys to a better life is improving the quantity and quality of your sleep.

In her book *Thrive*, Arianna Huffington says there are three simple steps we can take that have dramatic effects on our well-being:

Get just thirty minutes more sleep than you are getting now.
The easiest way is to go to bed earlier, but you could take a short nap during the day – or a combination of both. She calls sleep a "keystone habit," after Charles Duhigg's *The Power of Habit:* "Keystone habits start a process that, over time, transform everything...success doesn't depend on getting every single thing right, but instead relies on identifying a few key priorities and fashioning them into powerful levers."

Huffington said, for her, the most powerful keystone habit was getting more sleep. After that, she said many other things became easier and she accomplished more. This is truly an important and encouraging concept.

Move your body:
Walk, run, stretch, do yoga, dance. Just move. Anytime.
Don't sit too long. It's not good for cardiovascular health. Take breaks, and get up and move around. Sometimes when I'm at the computer for a while – and I spend hours there – I'll go downstairs and throw some clothes in the washer or dryer, unload the dishwasher, check for the mail, take a short walk or clean up in the yard. Not exactly model exercise, but it's better than sitting non-stop.

Introduce five minutes of meditation into your day.
Huffington provides a number of meditation techniques and their benefits. Overall, the important thing to do to be happier and increase well-being is to identify the proper things to do, then take action by forming the habits to do them regularly. In the *Prevention* magazine article "Infinity Man," super-inventor Ray Kurzweil includes some of his thoughts about living far out into the future and also reveals the regimen he follows. He said, "If I am well rested, I find that very few problems bother me."

Bragging About Not Getting Much Sleep

Sometimes people brag about how they get along on very little sleep and are still productive. The better question is how much more productive could they have been had they gotten more rest?

A well-regarded priest we had in high school said that the college crew team he was on was very good. He said their best rower was someone who drank and didn't keep himself in the best shape. However, since he was the best, he felt that he didn't owe the others any more. But the real question was how much better could they have been had he maximized his contribution by having better habits? Father said it would have made a tremendous difference in their team's results if he had. *Maybe getting more sleep could do the same for you.*

As a teenager, I'd fall asleep on the sofa, then wake up complaining to my mother about the time I wasted sleeping. She would say, "If you slept, you must have needed it." As I've gotten older, I've taken a nap on most days because afterward I felt more productive.

Taking a nap no longer than twenty minutes, and not too close to bedtime, can be helpful. If you frequently feel tired, the quality of your sleep could be the problem. See a physician who specializes in "sleep medicine."

If the doctor thinks you could have sleep apnea (when you wake yourself up multiple times during the night because of improper breathing or snoring), she/he may prescribe a "sleep study." They connect monitors to you to provide data about the number of times you may have apneas, and assess oxygen levels and other relevant factors. A sleep study can be conducted overnight in a health facility or you can be given a machine to take home. That's what I did the last time.

I've had four sleep studies done over the past twenty years or so. I've also gained some weight. That can contribute to snoring and breathing difficulties. An ear, nose and throat specialist told me that when her husband lost ten pounds, he stopped snoring, so losing weight might help. Drinking alcohol or having anything with caffeine in it, including chocolate, too close to bedtime can also interfere with sleep.

After each sleep study, the doctor recommended that I use a CPAP machine (Continuous Positive Airway Pressure) to improve the quality of my sleep. I'd have none of it. In return, I've had continuing sleep and snoring problems with resultant tiredness for years.

I had the fourth sleep study done recently through the University of Pennsylvania (Penn Medicine). The machine is greatly improved since the last one I saw: smaller, quieter, and less intrusive. I finally gave in. There's an adjustment to it, but I feel markedly better and not as tired or achy. My naps are not as frequent, or as long when I do take one. You might want to investigate it. It could make you feel a whole lot better and result in improved thinking and increased productivity. It might also help with pain relief.

Avoid Accidents

PEOPLE CAN "GO AHEAD OF THEIR TIME" IF THEY HAVE AN ACCIDENT. Look both ways before crossing streets. Stay off the cell phone when you do and when you're driving. Don't lean over to adjust anything when you're driving either. Keep your eyes on the road. Wear your seat belt. Make others wear them in your vehicle, too. Don't drive impaired by alcohol or drugs. Don't get up on ladders or a roof if someone more experienced can do it for you.

Many years ago, a former NFL receiver died in a fall from his roof, and he was a former professional athlete, probably still in far better shape than most of us. A reasonably athletic classmate was also injured when he fell from a ladder after only going up a few rungs. He was in a rehab facility for quite a while.

Home accidents can cause serious injury, too. Remove clutter in walking paths or on steps, hold railings when you go up and down stairs, be careful getting in and out of the tub or shower. (A famous, middle-aged Indian actor died recently when she slipped and hit her head on the bathtub.) Wipe up spills promptly. Don't touch electricity if you don't know what you're doing. Take small steps when walking on ice, and so on. Death is going to come to all of us. *What we don't want to happen to us, or to anyone else, are preventable deaths.*

Falls are a big risk. Dr. Atul Gawande, a noted neurosurgeon at Brigham and Women's Medical Center in Boston, says that the primary risk factors for falling are poor balance, taking more than four prescription medicines, and muscle weakness. People with all three risk factors have a hundred percent chance of falling.

Serious Health Decisions

IN HIS TRULY CLASSIC BOOK *BEING MORTAL: MEDICINE AND WHAT Matters in the End*, Dr. Gawande provides guidance for how we should make decisions when we have a life threatening illness, or when we are overseeing someone else's care. It's one of the best and most sensible books I've ever read. It's especially apropos to the life and death topics of this book.

Gawande says that families who have a loved one with a serious medical condition often ask him the same question: "Doctor, is there anything else you can do?" He says that *there is always something else that can be done. The question, though, is should it be done?* He says that a time comes when it is just better to provide palliative care, so that patients can enjoy whatever life they have left. He strongly supports beginning it as early as possible because it maximizes the enjoyment of life and frequently extends it. He also says that those who are ailing should have as much independence and control over their own lives as possible, ideally allowing them to live in their own homes until the end.

My aunt, who was a widow, suffered from a terminal illness. She was cared for in her home by her children who moved her bed to the living room of her two-story home. They rotated in shifts every night for months until she died. They did it with the grace and good humor they were brought up with. My aunt received the same loving care she extended to her husband, who was confined to a wheelchair for many years due to diabetes and an amputation.

About 30 percent of us will wind up in nursing homes. Most of us don't ever think it will be us. Some of us will be wrong. Sometimes it's unavoidable. But with more attentiveness, we may be able to prevent it or at least hold it off longer.

Dr. Gawande said that 63 percent of doctors overestimate their patients' survival time. The average estimate was 530 percent too high. *A very important factor for those trying to gauge the amount of time they have left to arrange their final affairs.* Better not to overestimate any remaining time. This makes a strong case for getting matters in order now. And when deaths are sudden, we get no notice at all.

Against All Odds

When someone gets a terminal diagnosis, Dr. Gawande's advice is prudent. At some point, it can become apparent that one's remaining life is likely to be relatively short. It's certainly reasonable to *ensure that all due diligence has been exercised* to determine if there are any reasonable options left.

I have two friends who came back against all odds. One had a cancer with only an 8 percent survival rate. He had surgery and went through three years of great difficulty. He's doing well today.

My classmate Jim Orr, from the Cincinnati area and former CEO of a major corporation and a member of the Board of Directors of several others, was given three to six months to live with a diagnosis of terminal liver cancer. He could have just accepted it, as I believe many would have, but decided to research all possible options thoroughly. He applied his skills of thoroughness and persistence that brought him success in life to researching a solution to the most critical problem he ever faced. And it paid off. After aggressive and innovative treatment, he ultimately received a liver transplant and is doing well now. Jim put it very well, "You have to be a full-time advocate for yourself when you're fighting for your life."

Jim's wife, Cathy, and other spouses and partners, have joined their loved ones in looking for solutions too. In some cases, more of the load falls on them because patients may not have the physical or mental strength to do it, or may be highly focused on their survival.

I pass on these examples so anyone facing a similar situation will know that sometimes keeping hope alive and being persistent can pay off. It's a personal decision each individual has to make, but it's important to know that you have researched all available possibilities and not just relied on local or regional advice.

I asked Jim to read my manuscript and to offer any insights he had about the subject. I have included them below as I felt his words are valuable for anyone facing this type of situation:

While death is something we cannot ultimately avoid, there are times when the effort to extend a quality of life, rather than surrender to death, is possible. I believe we are given the gift of life by a loving God, thus to give it up too easily, in a way could suggest we value it too little.

Fate or fatalism is a way of recognizing the inevitable or, in some cases, rationalizing our lack of control. Certainly life on this earth is finite. However, there are times when we may have more control than we might imagine. My own experience made me fully aware that although we may be presented with what sounds like a *fait accompli* with no viable option to return to a full life, what we do next, is a choice. Do we simply surrender this "gift" or do all within our control not to surrender too early what might actually be saved?

I cite here what happened to me as well as to my wife Cathy, at a later time. I want to provide my personal experience, not to suggest it could happen to everyone, but as a reminder that it can happen to some of us.

Two years after my diagnosis and one year following my transplant, Cathy was diagnosed with Chronic Lymphocytic Leukemia (CLL) and just weeks later with Cytomegalovirus so severe that she nearly died during a five-week hospital stay. After a week of 104-plus degree fever, multiple organs began to fail, and she was near death. The CLL impacted her immune system, but this major virus nearly killed her. The net of all this was after years of supporting me in my fight and fearing my death, she was now on her own journey and fight for the following couple of years.

This made me feel strongly about encouraging patients facing what may be regarded as a death sentence with no options, to fully explore the options that may be available to them. At a minimum, the exploration will leave them feel more informed.

The concept of aggressive advocacy is a critical consideration for all facing a potentially fatal outcome. It must be recognized that what is a certainty in the minds of some may simply be a high probability. This by no means suggests that all such exploration and efforts will always lead to a positive outcome, but in some cases it may.

From our experience come important lessons. I've listed below some of the key conclusions, which we offer not as a solution for everyone but as a checklist of things to consider when faced with a life-threatening illness.

These are clearly dedicated to providing the best chance to survive and thrive, but they are no guarantee because no one can give you one:

- Life is a gift from God, which is not to be easily abandoned.
- Death is inevitable, but not necessarily now.
- You must be your own advocate – you will find no one better.
- Recognize you may have more control than you think.
- Listen to many voices but make your own decisions. Surround yourself with those who love you and those who may be able to help. This includes family and friends, as well as physicians, including some who may not be treating you but may have some valuable insight, and others who may have been in a similar situation.
- Do your own research – there is a great deal of information and research on problems similar to yours. They may sometimes be discouraging, but it is important for you to know everything you can. The internet can be helpful, but you will often find incorrect, confusing, and misleading information. Stick to real research from accredited experts and institutions.
- Don't take NO for an answer. You may hear bad news and some may not give you any hope. However, that is not the time to quit.

–   Decide if you are willing and prepared to FIGHT for your life.
–   Ask questions. Physicians are typically well trained and very knowledgeable, but just like baseball players, lawyers, and other professionals they are not all created equal. Nor are they, or any institution, expert in every area of disease and medicine. Do your best to find one who is willing and capable to fight with you to beat your disease.
–   Make your own decisions. It is your life. You must decide what to do.

This is one man's opinion, but based on real-life experience. Some have said that my survival is a miracle, and that may be so. It was certainly described that way by many experts with extensive experience. At a minimum, it supports the belief, "That God helps those who help themselves."

To show their gratitude for being cancer free, Jim and Cathy made a major gift to help establish the James and Catherine Orr Endowed Chair of Liver Transplantation, which will benefit University of Cincinnati's liver transplant program. It aims to support research, medical training, and patient care efforts within UC's Department of Surgery.

We can all say thank you in our own special way, for the good things that have happened to us by helping to make them possible for others.

The Role of Physicians in
End of Life Decisions

DECISIONS LIKE THESE ARE ONES WE DON'T MAKE ALONE. WE DEPEND upon the medical opinions of physicians to guide us. Most of the time, we probably follow their guidance. Other times, we might decide to do something different. The role of physicians is important, nevertheless. In their "Top Doctors" issue, *Philadelphia* magazine featured "A Good Death," by Dr. Mary Kraemer. She is co-director of the palliative care team at Temple University Hospital. Her thoughts give excellent perspective and balance to what's already been mentioned:

"Physicians walk a fine line between being honest and being a source of possibility, of hope. It's easy to want to lean into the hope: It makes us feel good to give good news rather than face the hard truths. But when we doctors let go of the realities of illness, when we can't face the truth ourselves, we let patients and their families down, often when they need us most. [...] I help patients and families understand their circumstances, so they can make choices that are right for them. [...] We often keep pushing without knowing if our patients *want to keep pushing.* [...] Patients and families want to know what to expect, even if they're afraid to ask. They want to have time to prepare, to focus on forgiveness and farewells, and to define their own ending. [...] In treating end-stage disease, I see unfair things happen to people every day, but I also bear witness to remarkable love and resilience."

Dr. Kraemer explained to a patient that if she continued treatment, she would probably die in the hospital. When she understood that, she said she wanted to go home to be with her grandchildren, watch the birds at her favorite bird feeder, and simply watch life around her. "She was in charge of her life (and death) once more." She left full of hope and relief.

Whatever decisions we make for ourselves, it's that hope and relief we all want. There isn't a wrong answer. Just one that's right for you.

Competing Opinions About Facing Death

THERE ARE TWO COMPETING OPINIONS. THE FIRST, EXPRESSED BY Dylan Thomas in his famous poem:

Do Not Go Gentle into That Good Night

Do not go gentle into that good night,
Old age should burn and rave at the close of day;
Rage, rage against the dying of the light.

The second opinion is not to rage against it, but to embrace it.

We probably like to think that we would put up a fight, perhaps until the very end. Others may opt not to go through long and debilitating treatments, but to accept things and to enjoy whatever amount of "normal life" they have left. It's a decision we may have to make at some point. Do the research, take the advice and information you get, and decide what's best for you.

If at all possible, the person facing death should make the decision. Sometimes, others who are well-intentioned, including physicians, want them to keep getting more treatments and trying more possibilities. However, in one case I know, after already receiving many treatments, the person had had enough and basically said, "No more." That decision would have been made sooner had it been left solely to the patient. We all want to think that we have done everything possible for a loved one, but that has to be balanced with the patient's wishes and what they are being put through.

Don't Procrastinate – Put First Things First

MY UNCLE, MY AUNT'S HUSBAND FROM ABOVE, WAS A CAPTAIN IN THE New Jersey State Police, highly respected by everyone who knew him. He helped me many times when I needed it. I would go to visit him and my aunt occasionally. They were very gracious to me. When he was in the hospital, and I knew he was very ill, *I intended to go visit him. Just about the time I was getting around to doing it, he died. If you intend to visit someone who is ill, if they are able to have visitors and are open to it, don't put it off.* Even though I went to his funeral, it still troubles me that I didn't see him before he died.

In the same vein, my father used to say that "the road to hell is paved with good intentions." My friend Raman, a retired and learned colleague, who was our college's only Fulbright Scholar, laughed out loud when I told him that. He said his father used to tell him something similar when he was growing up in India: "If you are thinking about doing something good, do it before you can count to three." It's wise advice. Don't let life get in the way of what's really important. As Goethe said, "Things that matter most should never be put at the mercy of things that matter least."

Improved Thinking

IN *STUMBLING ON HAPPINESS*, HARVARD PROFESSOR OF PSYCHOLOGY Dan Gilbert makes it clear that our thinking, perspective, and predictions are often not as good as we think they are. It's an enlightening and humorous assist to helping people find happiness and making better decisions:

"We tend to overestimate the likelihood that good events will happen to us, which leads us to be unrealistically optimistic about the future. [...] We have an equally troubling tendency to treat the details of future events that we don't imagine, as though they are not going to happen. [...] The features and consequences we fail to consider are often quite important."

The old expression says, "What we don't know can't hurt us." Well, it can. We're probably not as creative as we might think either: "We think we are thinking outside the box, only because we can't really see how big the box really is. [...] We tend to compare the present with the past, even when we should be comparing it to the possible."

Avoiding regrets in life is very important, too: "People of every age and in every walk of life seem to regret *not* having done things much more than they regret the things they *did*." It's what I call "The Longest Rock" – rocking back and forth on a porch later in life *thinking of all the things you could have done, or should have done, but didn't.* Do things like that now when you still can, and you'll have fewer regrets later.

As a capstone to improved thinking, I highly recommend *Thinking Fast and Slow* by Nobel Prize winner Daniel Kahneman. It's challenging. Reviewing it is beyond the scope of this book, but it's very useful in recognizing errors in thinking and how different types of thinking and skills can be applied in different life situations.

Midlife Crisis and Improving
Our Circumstances

THE HAPPINESS CURVE: WHY LIFE GETS BETTER AFTER 50 BY JONATHAN Rauck says that the stress and dissatisfaction which can trouble us at different times of our life often eases off with age. We start feeling better about ourselves too.

Some of the lack of contentment might come from the realization that you aren't likely to progress organizationally to where you had hoped, that you have the feeling you're wasting your life, not achieving the dreams you may have had, or you find yourself mired in what many call a midlife crisis. Economist Hannes Schwandt called it: "that obnoxious sensation of being both puzzled and trapped".

One of the the book's major premises is that our life follows a "U-shaped" life-satisfaction curve. After a typical period of high satisfaction in our twenties and early thirties, there is a substantial drop off in "the middle years of adult life, that are often the most restless, stressed and unhappy." He points out that this is true "on average, not for every person." [...] "It's not an inevitability, it's a tendency."

Jonathan Rauch is a senior fellow at the Brookings Institution. He explores these and other facets of life in his well-researched and hopeful book. If you're fifty or over, it's a book you should read. It will explain what happens in this sometimes troublesome time frame. If you're younger, it will provide a preview of what may be in store for you. Knowing what's to come can forearm you to deal with it a whole lot better.

Rauch chooses the apt masterwork, "The Voyage of Life" by Thomas Cole to model life's passages. "The Voyage of Life" is a series of four huge paintings on *Childhood, Youth, Manhood, and Old Age* showing a figure in a boat, assisted by a guardian angel, passing through major phases of life. They are romantic and arresting works. Unfortunately, Cole didn't get to experience all these phases himself, but obviously reflected on them a great deal. He died at forty-seven, but left a great gift of contemplation on the passages of life most of us live long enough to sail through. The 1842 versions of these paintings reside in The National Gallery of Art in Washington, DC.

The author includes himself in the book as an example of the U-curve phenomenon. I could certainly see myself in it too, as I believe many of you could, asking questions similar to mine: Why didn't I get a Ph.D or a law degree? Why didn't I become a Dean (which I narrowly escaped becoming), or a more successful business owner? What happened to my "plan" to retire at fifty-five?

We're far from alone in these situations. Rauch says that about 80% of people have been affected by "optimism bias" – believing something is going to come true, which doesn't. Effectively, we aren't good predictors of what's likely to happen in the future. I remember reading this pregnant phase about our decision making: "And who was the only one present for all these possibilities envisioned and the decisions made?" It was each of us. Sometimes we're affected by uncontrollable, outside events, but for the most part, what happens in our lives is the result of what we did, and how well we did it, or what we didn't do when we should have done something.

Be careful what you wish for. As the old expression goes, "Lord, protect me from my dreams. They might come true". Value what you have and be grateful for it – a message Rauch stressed as a true help in finding happiness.

But for a few lucky turns of events, I could have been in deeper trouble economically and otherwise. I applied for a Dean's position many years ago. I was one of the two finalists, but didn't get the job. At the time, I was greatly disappointed. In retrospect, it was one of the best things that ever happened to me. For many reasons, I would have been wholly unsuited for it and probably very unhappy. The perspective of time tells us how fortunate we may have been –

something that is likely wholly unclear at the time.

Similarly, the pension fund I was required to join as a college professor many years ago, has become my largest asset. Other than steering it in certain investment directions, the fact that I have it was something I didn't do voluntarily, it was done to me. We're sometimes the beneficiaries of things we had little to do with.

"Midlife Crisis" is Not a Crisis

What is often called a "midlife crisis" Rauch says is wrong. "We need to understand why midlife satisfaction is, for the large majority of people, not a 'crisis', but a natural and healthy transition. [...] Some sociologists call this new stage of life, *encore adulthood.* (*Finding Meaning in the Second Half of Life* by James Hollis is a useful guide for entering this new phase of life.)

Rauch identifies that over time there is a change: "And often, seemingly as inexplicably as it had descended, the fog began to lift." When the rubber hits the road again and we have a more realistic view of what possibilities remain for us and we come to terms with it: "Emotionally we lower our sights and learn to settle. Settling increases our contentment."

This low period might sometimes call for medical intervention because it could be clinical depression. But Rauch says this is rare. Most often it's not "a mood disorder, but a *contentment disorder.*" Counseling can help with that or having suitable friends or mentors listen to provide perspective.

The author cites John F. Helliwell, a prominent figure in happiness economics, who quotes Aristotle: "Deeper satisfaction comes not from feeling good, but from doing good: from cultivating and maintaining virtuous habits that balance one's own life and create and deepen ties with others." Strong social ties are often cited in research as not only something that can better our lives, but also as a factor that can cause us to live longer.

Comparisons can also be detrimental to happiness. Rauch said that "Self-critical voices that pestered me about wasting my life insisted on comparing upward, which is the worst thing you can do. As Richard Layard, a pioneering happiness economist writes, 'One secret of happiness is to ignore comparisons with people who are more successful than you are: always compare downward, not upwards' ". If there is anything that probably causes us to be more grateful for our lives, making comparisons downward is probably it.

Rauck points to Elliott Jacques, a Canadian psychoanalyst who in "Death and the Midlife Crisis" (*The International Journal of Psychoanalysis*), wrote "The midlife crisis is a reaction which occurs not only in creative genius, but manifests itself in some form in everyone". [...] "In middle age we are forced to resign ourselves to all that we cannot be or do". [...] Important things that the individual would have liked to achieve, would have desired to become, would have longed to have, will not be realized."

The better news is that most people adjust to this realization and operate from an improved plateau. As part of the process, the greatly overused expression to "think outside the box" is often heard. The better approach is to realize that the box for you is probably much larger than you think:

"There are many more facets to us that the last role we played" – Betty Aberlin, Actor ,best known for her role as Lady Aberlin on *Mr. Rogers' Neighborhood*.

Factors in Determining Happiness

Your genes play a role in happiness too. We get about 50% of our immutable "set point" personality structure and basic happiness level from our parents. Research by Sonia Lyubomirsky confirms this in her book, *The How of Happiness*. Happily, some of the remaining portion is within our ability to influence.

Relatedly, Rauch indicates that Martin Seligman's previously mentioned *Authentic Happiness* offers a formula for happiness:

H=S+C=V where H is your enduring level of happiness, S is your set range, C is the circumstances of your life, and V represents factors under your voluntary control.

Rauch says we should add a "T" to that for "time", more specifically aging. Through their research, Andrew Oswald from the University of Warwick and David Blanchflower from Dartmouth University postulated that, "Age, all by itself, plays a role as a determinant of happiness." That provides hope for all of us in the future. If things are difficult, if you keep breathing long enough, your perspective is likely to improve, even if your situation doesn't.

Rauck uses examples of many respondents to his questionnaire who he subsequently interviewed. He mentioned Anthony, who at age forty-six, believed he had peaked. "His best personal growth and most exciting days are behind him, or so he thinks. He is very likely mistaken."

If you are thinking this way, maybe you are too, so have hope and keep moving forward. That sometimes means moving sideways too. Anthony said his passage was a "new normal"- "the last death of childhood". We learn to move forward to find a truer, and often highly improved, self.

Rauch also speaks of the "V-shaped curve" where one's life is going along well, but then takes a steep dive far below the U-shaped curve. We all make mistakes, but the message is to avoid the truly big ones because recovery from them can be difficult and sometimes impossible.

How Can We Help the Situation?

Develop a Proper Mindset
Jonathan Haidt, who Rauch identified as one of the world's most innovative thinkers, said he thought of his own life "much less as a project or city to be built, and much more as giving myself the right kinds of experience and exposure and letting time do the work." Rauch noted that "Voluminous research shows that the undercurrent that drags us lower normally does switch around the time you think it never will." Unfortunately, some abandon hope too soon, not realizing that substantive relief and improvement were close at hand.

Accept Life

The author asked his ninety-four year old neighbor Nora about what the key to satisfaction was. She said, "I would enjoy every day as it comes. Take what the day brings. Acceptance – and not worrying." The Bible says it well: "You worry all day and what do you have to show for it?" Akin to the ultimate acceptance expressed by the renowned Indian philosopher Krishnamurti: "I don't mind what happens."

Take Things by the Smooth Handle

This was one of Thomas Jefferson's "Decalogue of Canons for the Conduct of Life". Rauck asked his father how he was able to put anger issues he had earlier in life to bed. His father said, "I just stopped having five-dollar reactions to nickel provocations." Obviously, a learned art. I'm still working on it.

Take the Emphasis Off Yourself

Be kinder. Look for opportunities small and large to do it. Even if you're facing problems yourself, you can't always get help, but you can always give it. That helps someone else – and it will help you too.

Live in the Present

The past is over. The future isn't here yet. Focus on the present. It's what builds a better future. If the past is standing in your way, cognitive therapy can help to reframe matters and enable us to refocus on making meaningful progress.

Avoid Sudden, Risky Moves

Think things through. Sample if you can. Make "little bets," as Peter Sims says in the title of his book by the same name. Take some time to accumulate savings needed to make a successful transition. If the thought enters your mind to just quit your job, in most cases, it's probably far better to get good advice, plan, and take your time. And if you do go, it's better to exit professionally. Don't burn any bridges behind you. You may need to cross back over them later. I left a previous employer on good terms and was able to return almost five years later. A highly regarded engineer I knew was able to do the same in a very tight employment market. Rauck says, if you are going to move, "move laterally (into something that's related), incrementally, constructively and logically. That reduces the odds of impulsive mistakes and helps keep the downside manageable."

Be Patient

Sometimes it might be the time to take action and to make a change. Other times, it may be better to wait. Rauch says of the U-shaped trough, "*It gets better.* [...] "Waiting is a way of working with time and letting time work with us." Implied in this is having enough patience to let matters unfold without forcing the issue.

You're Not as Old as You Think

Think you're getting too old for all this? Consider the wisdom of Elizabeth, a member of a women's group primarily in their sixties. Rauch said, "She was eighty, not sixty-five, and she wanted to say that time was not as short as others assumed. 'You all sound like you think sixty-five is old because the world tells you sixty-five is old, she admonished. As a few years go by, you'll realize that sixty-five is pretty young."

Most people probably have more time than they think. Remember: *Plan to live to be one hundred.* Even if you don't, you can fill your time achieving goals *really meaningful to you,* for as long as you do live. That will give you a better and happier life.

Death Can Teach Us to Live More Fully

THE UNTETHERED SOUL: THE JOURNEY BEYOND YOURSELF BY MICHAEL A. Singer contains a great deal of wisdom about living your best life. The selected excerpts below include how contemplating death can give us a better life:

"Why wait until everything is taken from you before you learn to dig down deep inside yourself to reach your highest potential? [...] Death is not a morbid thought. Death is the greatest teacher of all in life."

"Everything is a million times more meaningful in that final week. What if you were to live every week that way?"

"Death changes everything in a flash. Maybe you should look deeper. Be willing to say what needs to be said and do what needs to be done."

"Learn to live as though you are facing death at all times, and you'll become bolder and more open. *If you live life fully, you won't have any last wishes. You will have lived them every moment.* There's nothing to take because you're already fulfilled."

But We Don't Need Death
to Give Life Meaning

In his *Prevention* article "Infinity Man," Ray Kurzweil says we don't need death to give time a purpose. "The things we can do with life – have relationships, be creative and create knowledge are what give life meaning." It's up to us to use the time we have by doing what is meaningful.

The next sections, "Growing Up in a Funeral Home" and "The Takeaway from Seven Decades," aren't meant to be downers, but to offer some details about funerals and funeral homes. The focus should always be on fulfillment, happiness, and finding contentment and peace. Put simply – living a fuller life.

The Need for Love

I DON'T WANT TO COMPLETE THIS SEGMENT ON HAVING A BETTER LIFE to end talking about death, but rather something that could increase our well-being and happiness. Love, in one form or another, is an obvious part of a happy life for most people. It can be the love of another person and the love we feel from others or a passion that might substitute for it, or augment it.

On the Swiss television broadcast "Passe-Moi les Jumelles" (Pass Me the Binoculars), an ornithologist spent his life in the pursuit of birds, photographing them and pursuing them as a hurricane chaser would. He said that he had effectively given up having a family in his life to engage in his pursuits. For him, that was his love. There are many other similar ones. For most though, it involves loving interaction with another person or other people.

I have not read Alain Botton's books, but they are highly rated by many readers. They provide insight into relationships and what can make them work and not work. I heard him interviewed on the PBS broadcast, "On Being" about his book, *The Course of Love*. He has a fascinating, and very helpful point of view. He says relationships don't usually fail because one or both of the partners are "flawed human beings", but more simply because of what happens in lives.

He's also a fan of gallows humor. He emphasized it saying that "we're all going to the gallows." It's just a matter of when and where. What we do between now and then (sometimes called the "the little dash in between" on a gravestone) is what we should strive to improve. The insights in the following chapters may help. One thing seems to be key: well-being and happiness come from focus on someone, or something else, not on ourselves.

"The little unremembered acts of kindness and love are the best parts of a person's life." – William Wordsworth

"What you are seeking is seeking you." – Rumi

"The greatest use of a life is to spend it for something that will outlast it." – William James

PART II

Growing Up in a Funeral Home

DEATH IS A TOPIC MOST PEOPLE DON'T WANT TO THINK ABOUT, BUT IF we're getting older, facing a serious threat to our life or are responsible for overseeing someone else's care, the more likely we are to think about it.

This is not to say that we always see it coming. A male classmate and a former female colleague spent the Christmas holidays with their families. By March they had died.

Two guys I grew up with died at twenty-two and twenty-seven. The first was in a drunken driving accident where he was a passenger. I helped my father lift him on to the embalming table. He wasn't the first of some of the guys I knew who I saw in the funeral home for the last time.

The other was my friend Al, a coach for the Marshall University football team. He was killed in the team's plane crash in 1970 that the film, *We Are Marshall,* was based on. We grew up together and went to the same grade school and high school. He and Ed, another good friend, were two years ahead of me in school. They were great athletes. We all lived about fifty yards from what was then St. Lawrence School in Lindenwold, New Jersey. We played basketball, baseball, football, and wiffle ball, and generally hung out. We played football on a lawn between the funeral home and the neighboring rectory. What a life! I owe both of them a great debt. They convinced me to go to Gloucester Catholic High School – one of the best things that ever happened to me. It was a horrible shock to see Al die so suddenly and in such an awful accident, leaving a wife and two young sons.

A friend of sixty years, one of Al's classmates, who was in apparently good health and also worked out regularly, collapsed without warning as a spectator at a sporting event. His organs were donated the following morning. He was as considerate in death as he was to everyone in life. One of our mutual friends told his sons that he was the person they should aspire to as a model of a good man. I felt the same way.

You can probably add to these, several more unexpected deaths. We don't all get advance notice. It's a strong reminder that we should enjoy life day by day and not put it off until retirement or vacation.

Sudden deaths are emotionally difficult on the survivors, sometimes financially too. In a way, an unexpected death is "easier" on the deceased since there was not much long-term suffering. Having life insurance to protect your dependents is of utmost importance – and typically the need far exceeds what is offered through the life insurance at work. Six to ten times one's annual income is often a recommended amount.

Those who pass from this world after extended pain and suffering find it more difficult, but in some respects, it may be "easier" on survivors because they lose someone piece by piece, rather than in a flash. This does not factor in the physical and emotional burden borne by long-term caregivers, truly among the angels of this world.

A World of Shared Experience

I'D LIKE TO TELL YOU THAT I HADN'T THOUGHT MUCH ABOUT DYING until I got older, but that would be a big lie. I grew up in a funeral home – with my father Tom, my mother Marge, and my sister Marianne. My mother was a nurse. Combined with my father being a funeral director, we had many conversations at our dinner table that seemed perfectly normal to us, but would have grossed out most people as "not polite dinner conversation". Subjects included autopsies, embalmings, blood, causes of death with all their attendant symptoms, jaundice, diseases affecting internal organs, combined with actually seeing them on a few occasions: "This is a liver. This is a heart. This is a kidney."

I also witnessed autopsies in progress a few times when I went to the hospital to pick up a body, drove bodies to another funeral home, helped my father with removals of the deceased from homes, carried caskets, helped to dress bodies, answered the door for floral deliveries in the afternoons, covered the door at viewings, set up and took down chairs, vacuumed the downstairs carpet in the funeral home, turned the funeral home lights on at night, emptied and cleaned ashtrays from the smoking room downstairs, next to the casket display room. I was a pallbearer, wheeled caskets in and out of church, and performed several other jobs that anyone who grew up in a funeral home could easily relate to and surely add a few more.

While the experiences mentioned in this book are often similar, I know many others who grew up in a funeral home probably helped more, and also saw more than I did. While I've tried to provide a picture of what it was like to grow up in a funeral home, I've also left some things unsaid as a matter of discretion and privacy. This is not a tell-all book. It shouldn't be.

In his book *Growing Up in the Mortuary: Thoughts on Death*, Richard Packham recounts some of his memories:

"My parents purchased a huge, old boarding house in an old residential district and remodeled it into Peck and Packham Mortuary in Blackfoot, Idaho. When I was sent down to fetch Dad for supper, I might interrupt him at work on a body, embalming it or dressing it or applying its make-up. Dad was a craftsman, proud of the quality of his work."

(This would have been a common sight for my sister and me, too. My father was meticulous and took pride in trying to do his best for the families he served. Idaho is a long way from New Jersey, but no matter how far removed in geography funeral homes are, there clearly is a commonality of experience.)

"I also helped (my father) dress bodies and lift them into the casket, especially if the deceased was a large man. Nowadays there are special derrick-like rigs that make the lifting easy, but my Dad just used his back, and mine."

(We had no such devices either, but I wish we had. My father did a lot of lifting. If Jack, who served his apprenticeship with my father, or I weren't available, he would lift the body himself or occasionally call upon one of two trustworthy neighbors to help him. Lifting bodies that are limp is not easy, no matter how little they weigh. Dressing a deceased falls into the same category.)

"When you grow up as I did, death loses some of its mystery and dread."

(That's certainly been true for me – especially the mystery part. I never had any dread. It has not stopped me, however, from feeling sad emotions and loss when those I cared about died. Even if you believe that you will see someone again, the fact is that you can't see them anymore now. You miss them and it hurts. Fortunately, for many people, acceptance and healing takes place over time. The person isn't forgotten, but it just becomes different. After a while, the cream rises to the top. The good memories help crowd out the sad ones. Unresolved issues are another matter. It's good to clear up any unfinished business while someone is still alive. Once they're gone, it may be difficult or impossible to do. You'd have to live with that. Sometimes that's not easy.)

"It's not grief over the death as such, but the realization that part of my own life is gone, never to return, the same sense of loss as when you think of long-gone, happy days, that can never be relived."

(Death reminds us of our own mortality, especially as we get older. We all have memories of happy days, and we carry them with us. It's not the same when those memories get interrupted by the deaths of those who were part of them. This applies especially to our parents. In a tribute given to his late father Howard Packham, Richard Packham quoted the words of Emily Dickinson, "Hold your parents tenderly, for the world will seem a strange and lonely place when they are gone." I've found that to be very true, too.)

Marianne and I witnessed many sad things growing up. But it wasn't a constant downer as some might expect. You'd have to be made of stone though, not to be affected by some things that we saw. Similar things have happened as I've gone through life, as they have for most of us at one time or another. As a healthcare chaplain working primarily with Alzheimer's patients, Marianne, like my mother, has seen many patients weaken and die. She is one of God's angels on earth, lending a kind and patient ear to the needs of others, something our mother was renowned for.

Funeral Calls and Removals

If my parents or Jack weren't at home, Marianne or I would answer the phone: "Good Morning, Danks Home for Funerals." My father trained us to take down basic information if someone called in with a funeral:

- Name of the deceased
- Address of the deceased
- Telephone number
- The name of the person calling
- Is the body at home or in the hospital?
- Has the body been released by the medical examiner?

Subsequently, my father would contact the family and arrange to remove the body from the home or the hospital. He was a strong believer that when someone called his funeral home, they wanted him personally. That's how he conducted his business. Today, it wouldn't be uncommon for other funeral home staff to make the call to the family and to make the removal. In busier funeral homes, this is a necessity. No one could do it all. And with the advancing age of the funeral home owner, it's sometimes sensible to have younger staff handle some of the more strenuous tasks.

It was not uncommon for removals to be made at night. On a number of occasions, my father would wake me up and tell me to get dressed. I'd clean up and put on a suit and tie. In the meantime, my father would shave and put his suit and tie on. Then we would drive to the home promptly, which usually was local.

My father would speak with the family privately. Then with just the two of us present, I would help him place the body on the stretcher. We would cover the deceased carefully with a sheet and a thick gray woolen blanket, then strap it to the stretcher very securely and carry it to our conservative, black station wagon. (This was the forerunner of minivans that are often used today for the same purpose.)

Once we got back to the funeral home, I'd help my father lift the body on to the embalming table. I was fairly sizable for my age, so the lifting was never a problem. I would go back to bed, but my father would begin embalming the body immediately. This could take several hours, depending on the circumstances. He felt that there were fewer problems with the embalming when it was done promptly.

A further consideration in doing the embalming immediately was that my father did not want things to back up. After making a removal during the night, he may have had a funeral a few hours later that morning, and possibly also had to make arrangements with a family for another funeral in the afternoon. Sometimes while these things were happening, another funeral would come in, so it made good sense to complete the embalming promptly, so that it wouldn't be put on hold. It never was.

One removal I remember in particular was at the convent next to our grade school. One of the elderly nuns died. I was always afraid I would get her for class. She was known to be tough and gave tons of homework. Somehow, I avoided getting her. It was a common fear of many students at our school that they would get her when the grade assignments were announced.

When we entered the room, Sister looked peaceful, not at all the threatening personage that students saw her as. I couldn't help but think about all the good she had done in her life. I remember carrying her body down steep, narrow stairs from the second floor and seeing the other nuns crying, perhaps not wanting me as a student to see them upset like that. I also couldn't help but think that it must have seemed like a misfit to them that someone they saw running around the playground was now in a suit and tie in the middle of the night in this private and intimate space with them at such a sad time. While I felt a little uncomfortable, it made me feel good that my father had enough confidence in me to know that I would act appropriately in that unusual situation.

I never talked about things like this at school with anyone, not only because I had the good sense not to, but also because both Marianne and I knew that my father expected us to always be circumspect about what we might say outside. Anyone who grew up in a funeral home knew better. Funeral homes, like doctors' offices, law offices, banks, and other similar entities should all follow the same rule, "What you hear or see here, stays here."

My Father's Routine

NEVER KNOWING WHEN HE MIGHT BE AWAKENED DURING THE NIGHT with a funeral call – which could be any night of the year – my father took a nap in the afternoon whenever he could. We ate promptly at five o'clock, so he would finish dinner in time to be able to go downstairs and get things ready for a viewing. The family would come about 6:30 PM and the public at 7:00 PM. My father greeted people at the door as they came in. This was a good way to ensure everyone received a welcome and that he had met them. On other occasions, Jack or I would perform the same function.

I do not want to overstate any modest contributions of mine. For three years, Jack, my father's apprentice, who I still think of as the brother I never had, performed these same functions far more often, as well as doing embalmings. Not having been licensed, that was obviously something I never did, but I saw plenty of them in the preparation room, where the washing of the body, embalmings and dressing of the bodies took place.

My Sister, the Embalmer

MY YOUNGER SISTER DID HAVE ONE EMBALMING TO HER CREDIT. WHEN she was in high school (the same one I went to), they had an annual Science Fair. She asked my father if it was possible to embalm a dog. As you might imagine, he had never done it before, but surmised that it would be possible, since for starters, dogs had circulatory systems too. So that became her science project.

A deceased dog was obtained from a local veterinarian and my sister, under my father's guidance, embalmed the dog. For anyone who knew her, she would be the least likely person to ever do this. The dog was respectfully displayed, with all appropriate scientific explanations of the procedure and comparisons between embalming a human being and a dog. The dog looked very peaceful lying in his little box, just as if he were taking a nap on the floor.

She got second place. I couldn't believe it. Someone who had a very nice presentation about space exploration got first place. In the sixties, space was big. Not to quibble, but I thought it was pretty hard to top the idea of a quiet, unassuming, Clark Kent-type high school girl embalming a dog. *That* was an original idea if there ever was one.

I believe there was some suspicion that my father had done the embalming for her, but he hadn't. My sister is as honest as they come. She wouldn't have been associated with something that wasn't on the up and up. Neither would my father. I was really impressed, though. She may not have won first prize but her project was as memorable as you could get.

Jack – Our Most Valuable Player

JACK MARINELLA, WHO SERVED HIS APPRENTICESHIP TO BECOME A funeral director with my father, was a true friend to me and our family. He helped all of us in many ways, especially in reducing the workload my father had.

Jack told me that high school would be the best four years of my life. In many respects he was right – lots of fun, free time, and great friends – and no responsibilities. It was good to have "an older brother." Jack took me to some of his semi-pro baseball games, which were a distance from the funeral home. He played first base and was a good hitter. After playing the whole game in the early evening, he'd drive me back to the funeral home. Then he'd have to drive about forty minutes to get home. He also coached our grade school football team. He drove me to pick up my date for an eighth grade dance and was a general advisor on what was "cool" and what wasn't. He was also a good dresser and drove a sporty, white and green Mercury. He did many things for me far beyond the call of duty. Basically, because of the kind of guy he was. He was well-liked and low-key with a good sense of humor and always highly respectful to everyone. He was also well known in the area where he started his business. It was one of the reasons he became an almost instant success.

Jack has owned a highly respected funeral home in South Jersey ever since completing his apprenticeship many decades ago. He's been supported in all this by his loving wife, Sandra. I went to their wedding about sixty years ago. They were a stunning couple.

Jack was in his early to mid-twenties when he was an everyday part of our family. He's eighty-six today. He was a wonderful blessing to my father and mother and to Marianne and me. He told me recently that he wouldn't have changed a thing about his life. He was very grateful for it all. He's mentioned many times the gratitude he has for my father, having taught him the training and operational methods he did, that helped him to succeed in business – especially the advice that he should go into business for himself.

It's good to know when the good we do is passed on. Jack has done that in his community. It is being continued into the future by his son-in-law and daughter, who continue the same tradition of caring and service that my father introduced Jack to so many years ago. I know Jack's success and caring for others pleased my father a great deal.

My Father, the Coroner

MY FATHER WAS ELECTED ONE OF THREE DEMOCRATIC COUNTY coroners when I was about ten or twelve years old. This provided additional income and also added to our already distinctive landscape. His reference books, with photos of various causes of death, gave me quite an education into some of the things he saw as coroner. Of course, anything I ever saw was next to nothing, compared with what police officers, firefighters, EMTs and medical examiners see regularly.

One of the guys I hung out with showed us a completely disrespectful photo on the cover of a well-known sensationalist newspaper showing a man who had been burned to death. It was even more grotesque than you might imagine. I thought it was faked. I was wrong.

In an ironic turn of events, his body came to our funeral home, through the coroner work I think. I helped my father lift him into a shipping case. This time at least, the paper wasn't exaggerating. The man's appearance was exactly what it was on the front page. (I've often thought of the caliber of the photographer who maneuvered himself into a house trailer to take such a picture, with total disregard for the man's dignity.) Because of his condition, it was not possible to embalm the body, so I watched as my father sprinkled a special powder on him for sanitary purposes. I felt sorry for the poor man and the suffering he must have endured. I only saw things like this occasionally, unlike my father who saw them more often. I think you get the idea by now. Being a funeral director isn't a snap.

Starting in Life and in the Funeral Business

MY FATHER GREW UP IN THE NICETOWN SECTION OF PHILADELPHIA, just below Chestnut Hill and Germantown. In his early twenties, he was a patient at St. Joseph's Hospital in Philadelphia. My mother went to nursing school there and subsequently was hired as a full-time nurse. That's where they met.

She was an outstanding student in high school and in nursing school. While she was at St. Joe's, she was assigned as the private nurse to care for Mother Katherine Drexel for a year. The since canonized Saint Catherine Drexel was a long-term patient there in the 1930s. Mother Catherine had a large inheritance – $180 million in today's terms – which she used especially to help the needs of Native Americans and African-Americans and to support other philanthropic causes.

Taking care of private patients, especially well-to-do ones, was considered to be a plum assignment because when such patients left the hospital, they often gave a substantial gratuity to their attending nurse. So the other nurses told my mother, "Blaese (my mother's maiden name), she's loaded! When she leaves, you're going to get a big tip!" The day Mother Catherine left, she gave my mother her sincerest thanks and two "holy cards" with pictures of saints and prayers on them. This was the second story I told at my mother's funeral. As my father frequently said, "Never count your chickens before they're hatched!"

My father was an excellent student. He started his career at Eckels College of Embalming (later Eckels College of Mortuary Science). He told Mr. Eckels he wouldn't be able to return for the second part of the one-year program because he wasn't able to earn enough to pay the remaining tuition. Mr. Eckels told him, "Thomas, you're a good student. You come back and finish and pay me when you can." And of course, he did both. An example of how much difference others can make in someone's life. My father often said he was forever grateful to Mr. Eckels for his kindness in helping him get started in life. It's good to help others in critical situations when we can. It can turn lives around.

When my father first started in business in the early 1940s, my mother worked the night shift for ten years as a supervising nurse in the county mental hospital. She also did the hairdressing for the deceased women who came to our funeral home, unless there was an outside hairdresser engaged or a family member wished to do it because, "I know how to do my mother's hair."

A colleague told me that her mother used to do women's hair for a funeral home. She always requested a photo, so she could see how the woman did her hair. It's a good idea to furnish one to the hairdresser if you have one. This not only makes the person look more like themselves, but it also avoids the family coming in at 6:30 on the night of the viewing saying to the funeral director that their mother never wore her hair like that. One way to avoid that is to have a female family member come to the funeral home earlier in the day to ensure that the hair looks the way the family expects it.

My parents didn't have it easy getting started financially. As a small boy, I remember very well my mother saying prayers with us before we went to bed. It regularly ended with, "God bless Mommy, Daddy, Larry and Marianne. Please send Mommy and Daddy business." That gives anyone an idea how tough it was to get started in the funeral business – both then and now. It might sound like a strange prayer, but it was one for survival. My parents certainly weren't praying that anyone would die, but just that when it did happen they might come to us.

My father was a good teacher. He generated additional income by running small group and individual classes to tutor those serving their apprenticeship to prepare to take their State Boards – the licensing examination that had to be passed in order to become licensed as a funeral director. He tutored Jack, too, as part of his apprenticeship. Later in life, he taught Medical Terminology classes for several years in a local hospital.

One of the men my father tutored, Jim McGuinness, and his highly supportive and loving wife, Marie, became lifelong friends of our family. They were great cheerleaders for me throughout my life. I loved them dearly. Until a few years ago, they were some of the few people who knew me from birth. I always thought of them as second parents. They have both since passed on. They had one of the most successful funeral homes in our area, built on their strong local identification with their beloved city of Woodbury, New Jersey, the strength of their character and their truly winning personalities and unparalleled sense of humor.

Propriety and Gentility

THOMAS J. DANKS PREFERRED THE TERM "FUNERAL DIRECTOR" TO "mortician". He thought that sounded too morbid. It wasn't uncommon in Philadelphia, where he grew up, and in our South Jersey area to "call the undertaker" when someone died. That was a common euphemism for a funeral director. He didn't care for that much either.

There was a local bar, located just down the street from the funeral home, which we could see easily out our front windows. I saw guys going in and out of there all the time, especially after work. When I was about nine or ten, I asked my father, "Daddy, why don't you ever go down to the bar?" He said, "When someone's mother or father dies, they don't want to have them taken care of by someone who sits next to them on a bar stool." That made a lot of sense to me – even as a young kid. My parents were very wise.

In the same vein, Marianne remembered Daddy saying he never wanted anyone to smell alcohol on his breath if he had to go out in the night to make a removal. Consequently, never knowing when a call might come in, other than perhaps a very small glass of wine on Christmas Day, he didn't drink during the time he was in business. And even in his retirement, he drank modestly.

My father was friendly and caring, but low-key. He had a strong sense of propriety that the community appreciated and respected. My parents' participation in many church and community activities helped them get better known and built confidence in the business over the years. There were already other local funeral directors who were established long before my father, so like many other businesses, he had competition. Few people could do what my father did as well as he did it. He was a true gentleman and very well-respected by anyone who knew him.

My Parents' Faith

MY PARENTS HAD GREAT FAITH. THE CATHOLIC CHURCH WAS ABOUT thirty yards away. They both went to daily Mass in the morning and sometimes again in the evening. They didn't wear it on their sleeves in the least. They showed it in the way they treated people.

Occasionally, we would have a body come to the funeral home through the coroner work. The county would pay for someone's very modest burial. A few times my father said there would be no viewing because no one would come. As a boy, I found it hard to believe that someone would die and no one, at all, would come. But it happened more than once.

On those occasions, my father and mother would take Marianne and me downstairs. We would kneel on the floor together in front of the casket and say the rosary for the person. (For those unfamiliar with this devotion, the rosary is about a twenty minute series of repetitive prayers said by moving one's fingers around beads as the prayers are said.) It is a traditional devotion for Catholics, but it can be mind-numbing if one lacks focus. My sister was as dutiful as always. But I surely wasn't, slouching down, complaining and getting tired – even though it was only about six-thirty in the evening. Only in retrospect did I appreciate how good my parents were to do this. In doing so, they also set an example for Marianne and me. Anyone who knew my parents would not be surprised in the least that they would do something like this because they did many charitable and caring things for others during their lives, related to the business and generally.

The Importance of Humility

IN SPITE OF THEIR ACCOMPLISHMENTS, COMPARATIVELY DECENT income for a small town, and the respect they had in the community, my mother and father were very humble.

Many of our caskets came from a local casket company in North Camden, across the Delaware River from Philadelphia. Many of the caskets were handmade. We were all great admirers of the casket company owner. This is an excerpt from a LinkedIn post I wrote about him:

Humility and Success Starting Small – "John, the Casket Man"

A model for me of thinking small, becoming successful, and staying humble with it all was a gentleman, frequently referred to in our house as "John, the Casket Man." I helped both my father and Mr. John Sandor carry caskets he made down into the casket display room. (When we had a funeral, Jack or I would help my father carry a casket up to the funeral parlor.)

Mr. Sandor came from the former Czechoslovakia to North Camden, virtually penniless, where he began making wood caskets by hand. He was a master with wood and with finishing it. He pulled a small express wagon across the then Delaware River Bridge (now the Ben Franklin Bridge) to Philadelphia to buy wood to make his first casket – just enough wood to make one casket, because he didn't have enough money to buy any more than that. He repeated this process over and over, until he was able to buy larger quantities of wood locally. From that very small beginning, he built the Camden Casket Company. He made the caskets, his wife sewed the linings, and his children were taught to help. They later followed in their parents footsteps.

Mr. Sandor was very kind to me when I was a boy. I think fondly of him. My father would frequently compliment him on his work and on his rise to success. He never changed. He would just get very sheepish about it all, in the humblest way you could possibly imagine, and in broken English he would make some self-effacing remark about himself.

He later moved his business to a suburban part of Camden County, where he located in an industrial park and built a beautiful home for his family with his own hands. That residence is now a professional office. I think of him every time I drive past it. After his wife of many years died, he died about two weeks later. He made his mark here in many ways, especially on me, because he started small and succeeded, and was a model of humility to emulate.

Getting a Share of the Business

SOMETIMES PEOPLE SAY THAT A FUNERAL DIRECTOR HAS A GUARANTEED business because everybody has to die. That's true, but they don't have to come to your funeral home. Like any business, a funeral business takes time to build. Obviously, because of its nature, it can't be promoted by any type of garish or insensitive advertising. It requires far more subtlety. In many respects, the funeral director represents the brand.

A high visibility location is very important to a funeral home. Close location to nearby houses of worship can also be helpful. We lived next to a Catholic rectory and what was then Saint Lawrence Church was next to that. (I was named after the parish. There were already four Thomas' in the family. My father thought that was enough.)

My father and mother knew the pastors and the other priests well. It was a blessing for me to know them as my neighbors. They were good men and very kind to me. I was an altar boy for three years, so I got to know them all. I was similarly blessed by the priests I had at Gloucester Catholic, as well as by the good Dominican nuns whom I had in both grade school and high school. They all made many sacrifices to serve a higher calling, set a good example for us and helped us learn and mature. Looking back on it, that was a tall order for them.

Good relationships with clergy, doctors, nurses, police, and fire officials are important to funeral directors because they make recommendations to families when they don't know where to turn when there is a death in the family.

Regarding having good relationships with local clergy, one of my boyhood chores was to bring in the trash barrels and the garbage can after pickup (also referred to in earlier days, at least in the Philadelphia area, as "the swill bucket" – in an era before

77

garbage disposals were common). I often needed my father's regular reminders to bring both in after they had been emptied.

The first pastor I remember was an older man with stark white hair, who was very direct and didn't have the best disposition. My father told me that one Sunday from the altar, as part of giving his sermon about charity, the pastor said, "Wouldn't you think that 'my neighbors' would bring in my empty swill bucket?" I should point out that we were his only neighbor. The church was on the other side of the rectory and a street was next to that. Nevertheless, my father was able to have a reasonable relationship with him, and fortunately very good ones with the other assistants who were kind to my parents when they were getting started in business.

Referrals from others who have already used a funeral home are important. Most important is getting repeat business from the same or the extended family (burying in the same family). If a funeral director has buried someone's father, and the family was satisfied, they are highly likely to use the same funeral director again.

Race and ethnicity can influence the choice of a funeral home. In the past, many families tended to choose a funeral director based on ethnic background, that is, Polish families would be inclined to take the funeral to the "Polish funeral home" in their neighborhood and Irish families would go to "the Irish funeral director" in their neighborhood, and so on. This was especially common in urban, ethnic neighborhoods. There is much less of that today.

In the Jewish community, a family typically selects a "Jewish funeral home", principally because they are familiar with religious requirements and cultural customs. Most African-American families also go to an "African-American funeral home." As a result, most funeral directors don't have many, or any, Jewish or African-American funerals. This is all fairly well recognized by everyone simply as a matter of personal choice by the families.

Who Decides Which Funeral Director?

It is the right of the next of kin to determine which funeral director to use. If there are disputes about who has the authority, legal assistance and the determination of a court might be necessary, but that would be rare.

The fact that a coroner or someone from the Medical Examiner's office, who is also a funeral director, has reason to be on the scene gives them no automatic right to take care of your loved one. It's up to the next of kin to make that determination.

It is also up to the next of kin to determine what funeral service, merchandise, and funeral arrangements they want. As part of providing good service, funeral directors may make recommendations, but any time a family feels pressured by a funeral home to do something they don't want to do, they should go elsewhere.

It may sometimes make sense to try a newer funeral director, if it is someone in whom you would repose trust and are open to other options for reasons of economy, modernity of facilities, or for other reasons. If you don't have any previous experience with the selection of a funeral home, ask for advice from those who know them personally or who have dealt with them before.

My father was "the new funeral director" at one point a long time ago. His demeanor, location next to the Catholic Church, and my parents' connections with the community all helped them progress from a funeral home with a very modest number of funerals, to the point later where the business became established.

The Medical Examiner's Office and Autopsies

New Jersey has excellent information from the NJ Medical Examiner's Office about the role of the Medical Examiner and autopsies at: www.me.nj.gov/faq.html

I've copied and briefly summarized some of the information. For further details, please visit the webpage directly or contact your county or state's Medical Examiner's Office. Your county government officials or your local police department can advise you how to contact them. All states have similar regulations in the public interest.

What Does New Jersey's Medical Examiner System Do?
In New Jersey, when a person's death is unexpected and the cause of death is not immediately known, the death is investigated by a Medical Examiner. The Medical Examiner also investigates deaths that are the result of violence or injury and deaths that occur in legal custody.

What do I do when a family member dies?
Call your local emergency number. The police and emergency personnel will respond. If there is a medical history for chronic disease, and there is nothing to suggest any other cause of death, the doctor who was treating the deceased will be contacted. The treating doctor is obliged to pronounce death and to issue an appropriate death certificate.

If a Medical Examiner investigation is warranted, the body will be taken by the Medical Examiner. Upon conclusion of the Medical Examiner's investigation, the body may be released to the funeral home of the family's choice. (Funeral directors determine whether the body has been released as a matter of normal course.)

What happens during an investigation?
During an investigation the Medical Investigator gathers information from family members, witnesses and others, and from the
death scene. The investigator works with police in analyzing the
death scene and also obtains pertinent medical records. The facts
may allow the medical investigator to close the case and refer it to
the family physician to sign the death certificate. The circumstances may require that the body be moved to allow for a more detailed
examination. This may involve an external examination (viewing)
or may involve a complete autopsy.

Why are investigations necessary?
Whenever a death occurs under circumstances that raise a public
interest, it needs to be explained and its cause and manner deter-
mined.

Autopsies are sometimes performed for reasons of public
health. For example, to protect the public, an autopsy may be
conducted to determine if a contagious disease is present. (On a
few occasions, our family had to take preventative medications in
response to this.) Autopsies are also conducted for public safety
and for the administration of justice.

Unnatural deaths are identified and investigated, leading to
proper classification for accidental death benefits. In criminal
cases, the investigation provides for proper evidence identification
and collection, leading to successful apprehension and criminal
prosecution.

What is an autopsy?
An autopsy is an external and internal examination of a body.
Licensed physicians, specifically forensic pathologists, acting as
medical examiners, will perform forensic autopsies to determine
cause and manner of death. After examination, the body is closed.
Specimens of body fluids and tissues are retained for diagnostic
testing however and, where necessary, an organ, such as the brain
or heart, may also be retained for further tests.

None of these tests will prevent the body from being released to the family for funeral arrangements. The autopsy will not interfere with funeral viewing. Autopsies are not always necessary, but in certain circumstances may be mandated by law. The law requires an autopsy in deaths involving a homicide, occurring under unusual circumstances, posing a threat to public health, involving inmates in prison, or when children die unexpectedly.

Funeral Directors' Services

IT'S PROBABLY GOOD THAT MOST PEOPLE DON'T KNOW WHAT FUNERAL directors do in too much detail. Part of their job is to make it that way, so that the pain of family and friends is minimized. That's all part of being a good funeral director.

It is a unique combination of technical skill, being a friend and confidant, being trustworthy, and having an opportunity to show true concern for people when they are at a low point in their lives. There are those who take advantage of the situation to prey on people at their most vulnerable time. Fortunately, they make up an extremely minimal percentage of practitioners.

There has also been an increase in regulatory protection provided to the public when dealing with funeral homes, including, but not limited to, itemizations of charges and providing required disclosures, as well as the availability of a state Mortuary Board where complaints may be filed if necessary. Always contact the funeral home owner first, to bring anything to his/her attention. Often, that will resolve any issues.

Confidentiality is extremely important in the funeral business. Funeral directors learn many things about relationships, financial status, and other private matters that any family would expect to be kept confidential. Anyone who is aware that a funeral director has breached that trust through gossip is surely one to be avoided.

Pre-Planning Funerals

FUNERALS COST THOUSANDS OF DOLLARS, SO PLANNING IS SENSIBLE. Pre-planning a funeral can help reduce the expense. Funeral directors like to pre-plan funerals because it shows a serious intention of the family to utilize their services in the future. Funds expended for prepaid funerals would be deposited into an escrow account. The money would be returned, with interest, upon request. Some states provide a guaranty fund to protect funds from misappropriation. In other states, trade associations perform a similar function.

An example of trade association protection is offered by The New Jersey Funeral Directors Services, Inc.:

"Once your funeral arrangements are complete, your funeral director will provide you with an itemized statement detailing your charges, along with your prepaid trust agreement. A check made payable to the 'New Jersey Prepaid Funeral Trust Fund' will be required at that time." A minimum deposit is required. The balance can be paid over time.

The funds are placed in an FDIC insured account for safety. Funds stay in your name and are completely refundable. Since 1981, over 47,000 consumer accounts are administered through more than 600 New Jersey funeral home locations. Speak to a local funeral director or to your state's Mortuary Board for further information.

Like many other expenses, funeral costs are only likely to rise in the future, so doing something about it now to reduce them makes sense. Selecting from options reviewed by the funeral director can also help reduce costs. Cremation is one of the major ways to do that. More on that later. It's a good idea to compare cost estimates from several funeral homes as they can vary, sometimes significantly. However, a variety of considerations, other than cost, should be factored into the decision, including satisfaction with the previous services of a funeral director.

Home Funerals

HOME FUNERALS ARE LEGAL IN EVERY STATE. NINE STATES REQUIRE THE assistance of a funeral director: Connecticut, Illinois, Iowa, Indiana, Louisiana, Michigan, Nebraska, New York, and New Jersey.

Burying someone "in the back yard" is another matter. In most jurisdictions, zoning and other laws and regulations would prevent it. It would be extremely unlikely that it could occur in any urban or suburban area. There are also requirements for how long an unembalmed body can be held prior to burial for health reasons. Today, some would also have questions about where cremated remains may be buried or what requirements there may be for their handling. Complete details on legal requirements regarding transportation of the deceased, funerals, and burial requirements are available from your state's Mortuary Board.

In the past, even though a burial may have taken place in a cemetery, or the body was cremated, some viewings were held at home. This is uncommon today. It caused practical problems for the funeral director having to move equipment and the deceased to the home, typically into a space that was far too small. While the sentiment of a home viewing was certainly understandable, it was impractical for many reasons, including waiting lines outside and inadequate facilities.

Funeral Expenses

IT'S IMPORTANT TO USE GOOD JUDGMENT WHEN DECIDING WHAT TYPE of funeral to have. People should plan their own funerals, whenever possible. That eliminates potential problems and arguments among family members. My parents planned their own funerals. It simplified matters for my sister and me. Funeral directors help with this since many people wouldn't know what considerations would go into the process.

Families want a loved one's funeral to be respectable, whether it involves a burial in a cemetery, a cremation, or donation to science. If a casket is selected, it doesn't have to be the most expensive one. Do what's reasonable and don't let emotions get the best of you, even if someone else is goading you. Go elsewhere if you feel pressure from the funeral home.

The funeral director will review an itemized list of expenses, so that you know what you will be paying for in advance and can also decide what expenses you might wish to eliminate, such as for livery (funeral cars to carry the immediate family and flower cars). It's not uncommon today for families to just use their own vehicles. The funeral home will transport flowers to the gravesite, or to wherever the family directs locally, whether a flower car is engaged or not.

Newspaper obituaries can be expensive. If expense is a consideration, run a brief obituary directing the public to the funeral home's website, where more detailed information can be obtained. Because of the expense involved in running obituaries, many have become shorter. That's unfortunate because they can provide a fuller picture of the deceased and her/his life.

Cemeteries add to funeral expense, not only for the cost of the grave, but also for opening it when the time comes. If someone wants to be buried in a cemetery, it's wise to purchase plots in advance, since the cost keeps rising. Cemeteries can fill up too, so if you have an interest in a particular one, or you want to keep your family together, don't wait too long.

Monuments and grave markers are also an expense. My parents wanted something modest, so that's what we did. Others feel differently about this. It's a good idea to do some comparison shopping and also to follow any wishes the deceased had.

The Critical Importance of Having a Will

A WILL IS A LEGAL DOCUMENT THAT DIRECTS WHERE YOU WANT YOUR property to go, and how other matters relative to you are to be handled, after you die. It has no effect while you're living. In addition to dealing with the distribution of your real and personal property, it may also specify whom you would wish to take care of any minor children you have. Such designees should always be asked if that is acceptable to them in advance.

When someone dies without having a will (dying intestate), the laws of the state will determine how assets are to be distributed. This might be wildly different than what the wishes of the decedent would have been. So if you want your property to be distributed the way you want, it is critical to have a properly drafted will in conformance with the statutes of your state.

In order to save a few dollars, or for other reasons, people sometimes decide to write their own wills or use some standard form they obtained. If such documents are later ruled to be legally invalid, the decedent's property will be treated as if she/he died without a will. Being dead, obviously there would be nothing the decedent could do about it.

Several factors could cause your will to wind up being declared invalid, such as the failure to have the proper number of witnesses required, lack of notarization of the document, notarization in the wrong place, or having contradictory statements contained in the document. It is far better not only to have an attorney draft your will to ensure that it is done properly, but also because there are other legal matters relative to this that you can be advised about, so you can make the appropriate decisions.

A highly experienced attorney, who is also a classmate and life-long friend, advised me on these matters. He also told me that non-attorney drafted wills typically wind up in court, where they are often ruled invalid. In any event, that process would add both time and significant expense to the process of having an estate settled. It is far better, and far less expensive, to simply do it properly in the first place by going to an attorney.

For those who insist on doing it themselves, at the very least, the testator (the one expressing his/her wishes in the will) should schedule a consult with an attorney to ensure that it meets the requirements of statute. However, consults would cost something too. The cost of preparing a simple will would very likely not be much higher than the cost of the consult, so why not simply have the attorney do it all, and know it is done properly in the first place?

Having a will is very important. It is one of those things that are like dentist appointments – often put off until later. One way to get it done is that anytime you need to see an attorney – for anything – such as for assistance in preparing a living will, discussed below, or getting a lease or contract for the sale of real estate reviewed, make that the time that you ask the attorney to prepare a will for you, too. It will make things much easier on your survivors if you do. It will also give you the peace of mind knowing that you have met your responsibilities in taking care of the needs of those who are im-portant to you – while you can still do something about it.

Having a Living Will –
An Advance Health Directive

A LIVING WILL IS A DOCUMENT THAT ADDRESSES WHAT WE WANT DONE with us medically during what could turn into our final illness. A living will does not have to be prepared by an attorney. Standard forms can be obtained through outside sources. My attorney recommended "The Five Wishes Program" (www.fivewishes.org) as an excellent source. It is a website you should visit.

Five Wishes provides a form, free of charge, which allows you to express:

- The person you trust to make decisions for you
- What types of medical treatment you would want – or not want
- What is most important for your comfort and dignity
- What important spiritual or faith traditions should be remembered
- What you want your loved ones and healthcare providers to know about you

The form provides excellent information about matters that you would need to make decisions about. While it can be done without legal assistance, a better course of action is to complete the form as best as you can, then take it to an attorney for further assistance and guidance about how to best answer the questions and what legal ramifications may be involved. I recommend having an attorney prepare the living will for you. He/she can use what you have already done, guided by the form, as a good starting point.

Here's some additional insight from the excellent article "Why You Need a Living Will – Even at Age 18" (Amir Khan, US News & World Report -12/19/14):

"A living will, also known as an advance directive, is a written set of instructions for how you want to be treated if you're no longer able to make decisions for yourself," says Mark Jordan, an estate attorney with Buechner, Haffer, Meyers & Koenig in Ohio. "It also appoints a friend or loved one as a health care proxy, someone who can legally make decisions on your behalf. It's meant to direct your doctors in a situation where the doctors cannot cure you and you can't tell them what you want."

The end-of-life-care-wishes discussion is not a comfortable one to have. But devoting time to it now can save everyone from experiencing discomfort, pain and anguish down the road. "Living wills are really an ounce of prevention that everyone should have after they have turned 18," says estate lawyer Donald Sienkiewicz, owner of Estate Preservation & Planning Law Office in New Hampshire. "Nobody, not your parent, spouse or child, can make legal, financial or health care decisions for you without a court order, unless you have delegated that authority to them in advance through a power of attorney or living will."

"For most people, living wills outline life support wishes," Jordan says. Some people also include a "do not resuscitate" order, (a DNR) which instructs doctors not to revive them if they stop breathing or their heart stops. When a person signs a living will, they're saying that if they're in a situation where their heart has stopped, here's what I want you to do. Two doctors need to make the determination that you won't recover before your living will kicks in, Jordan adds.

"One of the major benefits of having a living will is to spare your family the guilt of trying to guess what you'd want or from choosing options you would not have supported but that ease their anguish – in other words, prolonging your life so you remain in theirs," says Jason Martin, an estate attorney with Martin Law Firm in Pennsylvania. "Without this document in place, family members are left to make decisions, which can not only lead to significant conflicts, but can also lead to feelings of guilt, remorse or anger. Having this document in place may also prevent a large financial burden on your family or estate, since remaining on life support for extended periods may lead to substantial medical bills and costs for your necessary care."

Do Funeral Directors Charge Too Much?

IT MIGHT SEEM AS IF FUNERAL DIRECTORS MAKE TOO MUCH MONEY. But as in other businesses, staying in operation costs money and requires a reasonable profit.

Funeral directors not only have businesses to support, but also typical household expenses. In the past, funeral directors frequently lived above the business for convenience. It also reduced their housing expense. Today, many funeral home owners have a separate residence.

Our living space above the funeral home was not spacious. The new owner, who now has been there substantially longer than my parents were, made everything more spacious and commodious through extensive renovations. Renovations are necessary in funeral homes to provide sufficient space for additional funerals and to keep pace with the competition, but it's also an added expense that must be recovered over time.

Funeral directors may sell their businesses at some point, but buyers are limited to those who have a desire and aptitude for operating their own funeral home. A funeral business might not be salable for a variety of reasons. A primary cause could be that it "doesn't do enough funerals" on an annual basis. That's a substantive component in determining how much someone is going to get for the business when they sell. If business isn't good, it could wind up primarily being a sale for the value of the real estate.

Expenses include the cost of the upkeep of the funeral home and grounds. Most often, they're sizable, so painting, siding, and roofing costs are considerable. The inside must be well-maintained, including replacing the carpeting and interior painting periodically. No one wants to have their loved ones buried from a place that is poorly maintained.

Being a funeral home of modest size, my father did a lot of work himself: cut the grass, planted flowers, pulled weeds, painted, and did general maintenance inside and out. Most funeral directors also have to pay for plumbers, electricians, and other skilled craftspeople when needed.

I did a small amount of the maintenance work my father did. Jack did a lot of it. I especially hated pulling weeds. I was advised frequently that my technique needed improvement. I painted the exterior of the funeral home once and also the neighboring rectory. My parents left plenty of time for me to play and to have fun as a kid. And I did – in grade school and in high school.

Multiple vehicles also need to be purchased or leased. Hearses and limousines are specialized vehicles. They are colossally expensive, even when purchased used. As you might imagine, such vehicles have to be new or very late models, to maintain the respectability that families would expect. At this writing, such vehicles run in the $80,000 – $100,000 range. Some funeral homes have dispensed with purchasing them because of their reduced usage. Smaller funeral homes typically would not own them. In both cases, families and the funeral directors would rely upon local livery services and rent vehicles on an as-needed basis. Being a funeral home of modest size, this is something my father always did.

Added to these are the general expenses of taxes and utilities. Insurances including comprehensive general liability, auto, health, and life insurance also have to be paid. Embalming fluid, cosmetics, funeral equipment, furnishings and maintenance supplies are further expenses.

To meet the expenses they face, in some parts of the country, funeral homes have generated other sources of income by having them serve as the equivalent of community centers that fulfill a variety of functions, not just providing a venue for funerals. If this is done carefully and tastefully, it makes sense from a business perspective to have some additional profit centers. The stability of the business benefits all concerned. It can help serve the broader community in a variety of ways and can also provide greater exposure for the business. It takes a major financial commitment and more spacious facilities, so it's something that most often would have to start from the ground up construction-wise, rather than being a renovation to existing facilities.

If you were to choose a funeral home, would you want to select one that's established and successful or one that seems like it's on the ropes? If it's successful, that means that the funeral director has probably been doing the job well, has a good reputation and is making a good income. As long as families are being treated fairly and with kindness and professionalism, I see nothing wrong with that.

Life in the Funeral Home

DOWN TIME THAT FUNERAL DIRECTORS HAVE IS SOMETHING THE public rarely thinks about. *Funeral homes don't have funerals all the time, but income only comes in when they do.* But all the overhead keeps right on coming, nevertheless.

Another aspect of the funeral business – what do you do with the non-funeral related time you have? Depending upon how many funerals a funeral director has, there could be quite a bit of it. That's not something everyone could handle well. Nor is caring for people who are grieving as part of your daily occupation. So there are some well-being and psychological considerations with being a funeral director, too.

If a funeral director only has a few funerals a month, which is very likely early on in their careers, it virtually mandates that they or their spouse or partner have additional sources of income. By the nature of what they do, this is often limited to such things as doing related trade work, such as embalming for other funeral directors, assisting on funerals at other funeral homes, working for local or county government, or for a government agency, and other suitable endeavors. As honorable as these occupations are, it wouldn't include working construction, being in retail, or anything like that. The public would question someone's commitment to their business if the extra work they did was wholly unrelated to the funeral business. It is difficult to get started in the funeral business too, unless someone buys an already established business – and that comes at a high price.

Paying for medical, retirement, and disability benefits can also be a real issue. It might take a spouse or partner, or the funeral director working outside the business to get fringe benefits.

As a further consideration, ask yourself if you would want to do this kind of work yourself and also be available 24/7? Most people would never choose being a funeral director as an occupation. Most people also do their work and go home and have their private time. Funeral directors not only have more obligations, as any business owner would, but also have to be on call almost all the time.

As much as people are loved during their lifetimes, it is the natural order of things to want to have the deceased removed from the home or hospital as promptly as possible to avoid further mental anguish. A deceased's being in a funeral home, to most people, is being in a safe and respectable place. That offers at least some modest degree of comfort to the family.

It's a strange thing about death. Even when we've known for quite a while that someone's death is inevitable, it doesn't insulate us from the shock we have on the day when it actually happens. It's still usually hard to believe.

My father took his work very seriously. When people called Tom Danks, ninety-nine percent of the time that he was in business, that's who they got – in person. Today, many funeral homes have answering devices at the door and answering machines or answering services for evenings, nights and weekends, so they can have more normal lives. While I didn't grow up this way, it's certainly reasonable to me that there should be an improved work-life balance.

Other than one occasion that my father's sister, my wonderful and fun Aunt Anne, watched my sister and me when my parents took a short trip to Florida, or took us on an infrequent family vacation when Jack watched the business for a short time, I never remember a time that either my mother or father weren't home with us when we were growing up. That gave my sister and me great stability. I've been forever grateful for it, but it didn't give my parents much of a break.

Mega Funeral Homes

WHEN A FUNERAL HOME IS DOING MORE THAN SIXTY OR SEVENTY funerals a year, extra staff is going to be needed. With a hundred or more funerals a year, or sometimes in the hundreds above that, it's a full-time daily operation that requires full-time help and a great deal of monitoring, expense control, accounting and tax advice, and management skill.

Speaking of truly large funeral homes, in *I'm a Fourth Generation Funeral Director*, Whitney Kimball says:

We have 17 funeral homes — my dad and three of his cousins are the four owners, and they each operate a separate division. So although we're one company, we operate day-to-day as four separate little companies. I work with my father, my brother, my cousin, and four other funeral directors, and together the eight of us run four funeral homes.

People get freaked out by the idea of taking care of the dead as a living, but I just think people really don't know any better. The job's more about the people who are still alive – really, most of my time is spent fielding phone calls and meeting with people, making videos, and printing paper goods [...] talking to newspapers and arranging military honors. [...] The actual preparation of the body is really only about 30 percent of the day.

(All very true. The general public's focus is on the obvious: the removal and preparation of the body, viewings, and funeral services, but there's more to it than that. Funeral directors perform many other services that are pretty much taken for granted. If families had to attend to these details themselves, they'd see that there is a substantial amount of additional work involved.)

Because the work (funerals) comes in at all times, there really is no end of the day. Last year, we did 499 funerals – so breaking that down, it's obviously more than one person a day, but some weeks we're beyond busy and other weeks we're slow and start looking for something to clean or organize.

(499 funerals in a year is a colossal number. Only a small percentage of funeral homes in the United States and Canada have that many funerals.)

It's all about serving the people and being there because, gosh, if my mom passed away I would want someone to come right then because it'd mean the world to me.

(Being there for support and consolation is an important role of a funeral director. Many families don't have much, or any, prior experience with intimate loss. The funeral director's support can mean quite a bit at difficult times like this. My father was a strong shoulder. So was my mother. It's part of what helped their business grow.)

Conspicuous Consumption

HIGHLY CONSPICUOUS CONSUMPTION IS SOMETHING FUNERAL DIRECTORS should avoid. People expect a funeral director to have a life, but when it seems grossly excessive, there could easily be a kneejerk reaction to think that it's coming from overcharging for funerals, when in fact it could come from good business management, prudent spending, savings, investments, or inheritances.

Market Research

IN THE EARLY 1940S AND 1950S, THINGS WERE LESS SOPHISTICATED, management wise. Market research is one example. I remember my father keeping a small notebook. He would look in the local newspaper everyday to see who died and record which funeral director got the funeral. From this modest system, he kept track of whether he was getting a reasonable share of the available funerals. There is no rhythm or rhyme to funerals coming in either. A funeral director might have five funerals in a week, then none for the next three – sometimes longer. That gets scary, and there's little someone can do to turn that around quickly.

It can be disappointing to a funeral director when they see that a family they have buried in before has gone elsewhere. While that could mean that there was some dissatisfaction, it's not necessarily so. A childhood friend of mine was recently buried from a funeral home that their extended family hadn't used before. The simple reason was that my friend had, at one time, lived right next to that funeral home and got to know the owner well. It was just an outlier. Of course, the funeral director who may have expected to get that funeral may not have been aware of these special circumstances and thought that they had "lost a funeral."

In a similar case, decades ago, I went to a viewing. My deceased friend's father just about apologized to me for not coming to us, since we knew them very well. But they had other friends too, and he and the funeral director also had a close political connection. These circumstances happen occasionally. Usually, as in many other businesses, you're not going to get all the business, but if everyone is doing the job well, they're going to get their share.

The funeral director my father bought the business from had six funerals in the previous year. Over time, my father built that up to over seventy, which was quite an improvement in a small community. He met and helped many people along the way. My sister and I were very proud of my father and mother and for the goodness and caring they showed to the families who came to us. Their faith carried them through life. It was also the greatest legacy they left us.

The Condition of the Body

ANOTHER VIEW FROM THE OTHER SIDE IS HOW THE VIEWING PUBLIC may sometimes comment on the deceased's appearance: "He doesn't look good," "She doesn't look like herself," "He's got too much makeup on," and so forth. What the public can lose sight of is that most of them remember the person upright and in good health. Many may not have seen the deceased for a while – sometimes for years. The ravages of illness, cancer treatments, weight loss, age, discoloration of the body, and the impact of accidents and other factors may require a funeral director to make cosmetic improvements, fill out sunken facial features, use wigs instead of natural hair, and employ additional techniques. Like many other skills, some funeral directors are better than others in having the deceased make the best presentation possible.

Sometimes it takes some creativity. In accidental deaths, a body might be turned around from the head at the left top position in the casket to the other way around, because there was damage to the side of the face that could show otherwise.

When my father was serving his apprenticeship, a man's body had been cut in half by an industrial accident. The funeral director said there was no way the body could be viewed. My father suggested that the deceased be sutured together. He did it, and the body was viewed.

If a funeral director says that it would be better if the viewing were held with a closed casket, take the recommendation. There's going to be a good reason for it. There are some times when the deceased may have indicated a preference for this too or only wanted the body viewed by the immediate family.

Similarly, if the medical examiner, a physician, police officer or firefighter says that *no one* should view the body, the advice should be taken. *It is far, far better to remember a person as they were than to insist on seeing someone, and then having that awful memory with them for the rest of their lives.*

I'd give similar advice for any identification of a body required for legal purposes. It's much better to have someone who knew the person *well enough* to make the identification, and not have it be done by someone with close emotional ties to the deceased. It is the medical examiner who must be satisfied that a correct identification has been made.

Cosmetic and Presentation Skills

THE COSMETIC SKILLS OF A FUNERAL DIRECTOR CAN BRING A GREAT deal of comfort to a family and friends. The more a person "looks like themselves" or "looks like they are just sleeping" can give everyone quite a boost under the circumstances.

Jack very aptly calls what the deceased looks like at the viewing "a memory picture." It's the last time the person is going to be seen, so it's important that she/he looks as good as possible. How the deceased looks is also going to be a reflection on the funeral director – even though sometimes it shouldn't be.

I went to a classmate's mother's viewing a number of years ago. Her mother looked terrific. I mentioned it to my classmate. She simply said that the funeral director was "the best." A few years later, my classmate was viewed from the same spot. She looked terrific too. I thought about what she had said about the funeral director's skill. She was reconfirmed proof of it. It was an unhappy irony. She was a wonderful person who had been through quite a bit medically and died suddenly while in the hospital awaiting treatment for breast cancer.

A dear friend's mother died. She was the epitome of graciousness and friendliness, and a model person. I thought the world of her. I remember being really struck by how natural she looked – just as if she were resting on the sofa. Looking as natural as she did, just underscored how natural she was as a loving person. I think it brought consolation to her husband, children and grandchildren. It gave me some too.

It can also cause the opposite effect when the deceased doesn't look as good. In fact, it can be a distraction to trying to come to terms with everything that's happening. *But sometimes in spite of a funeral director's best efforts, only so much is possible.* I've seen the condition of bodies when they come in. Almost uniformly, they look far better when viewed than they did on arrival, but in some cases, there is only so much that can be done. Funeral directors shouldn't be judged on things beyond their control.

The appearance of the body is enhanced when funeral directors pay attention to the details: clean, lint-free, well-arranged clothing, no blood on a shirt after the deceased has been shaved, clean hands and fingernails, no threads showing, making sure that the knot in a tie is tied correctly and comes all the way up, shoes shined, eyeglasses clean, any extraneous hairs trimmed, and so on. I've been to many viewings. Funeral directors do a good job on these details.

Living Above the Funeral Home

WE LIVED ON THE SECOND FLOOR OVER THE FUNERAL HOME – LIVING over the store, so to speak. As you might imagine, my sister and I would often get questions like, "How can you sleep in a house with dead bodies?" or "Aren't you scared living there?" When I would mention this to my father, his response was, "It's not the dead that people need to be concerned about, it's the living." Our reaction to this was similar to what someone's would have been living over a deli. My sister and I grew up with it, so we never thought anything of it.

It's not unique that someone would write a book about growing up in a funeral home. Searching under that phrase, you'll see that there have been a number of previous books and articles written. People seem to have a curiosity about it – although they're probably not ready to give up their own living situations to move into one.

Celeste Donohue, a comedian and writer, grew up in a funeral home in Philadelphia. Her thoughts mirror those of my sister and me: "People have asked me if I was scared growing up in a funeral home and the answer has always been no. It wasn't scary for any of us, because we never knew life without dead people. I always looked at the dead as though they were temporary guests in our house — and I guess they were. My dad always treated them with respect, so we followed suit. They were like guests I'd never met before but was completely comfortable around."

(Marianne and I were too. One thing that was brought home continuously to my sister and me by our parents was the importance of respecting the dead and their bodies and properly preserving their dignity, while providing whatever service could be provided to their family at a reasonable price. My father said many times, "The body is the Temple of the Holy Ghost." We all believed it and acted accordingly. Whether others share that spiritual view, common decency mandates that everyone deserves respect in both life and in death.)

Kate Mayfield also grew up in a funeral home in southern Kentucky. In her memoir, *The Undertaker's Daughter,* she said, "Our family lived quietly, as silent as the grave, on the floor above. The staircase led straight up to our living quarters and offered no door of comfort, no solid thing to shut us away from the funerals and visitations that occurred below."

(This reflected our living situation, except that we had a glass-paneled door with a sheer curtain over it at the top of the stairs. A lasting memory I have is as soon as that door was opened when we had a viewing downstairs, the fragrant smell of flowers just permeated the air. It all comes back whenever I've been to a viewing since or even to the famous Philadelphia Flower Show. Viewings often produced a colossal number of baskets and sprays. Today flowers seem less plentiful. They have also frequently been replaced by financial donations requested by the family to go to a worthy cause.

The "quiet" part is a common thread for kids who grew up in a funeral home. Noise made upstairs would be an immediate distraction downstairs at a viewing. Noise I made – my sister never made any – would get my father coming upstairs in a hurry: "Turn that damn television down!" or "Who was doing that jumping!" – as if he didn't know. Anyone who grew up in a funeral home would tell you things like this happened in their house too.)

"My father didn't try to hide death from me. My earliest memories of life were all about its end. He was responsible for creating strong images that I'm able to conjure in an instant, like the way he used to stand in front of a coffin with his mortician's makeup kit. I stood by him transfixed and awed that he possessed the knowledge and the talent to paint the finishing touches on the corpse's lips."

(My father and mother saw death as part of life and we were brought up that way. We weren't shielded from it in any way. I remember standing next to my father many times, too, when he was making cosmetic touches to the deceased.)

Susan Portelance from Winnipeg, Manitoba related her experience in "Life Lessons from Growing Up in a Funeral Home" (Canada's *The Globe and Mail*):

"My parents acquired the funeral home in Deux-Montagnes, Quebec. It was all I knew. But as I grew up, I began to realize my life strayed pretty far from the standard definition of normal. I've slowly come to appreciate the effort my parents made to keep my life as normal as possible for us."

(This was certainly true for my sister and me. It never felt abnormal to us, in spite of what everyone else may have thought. My parents did a good job creating a home for us, even though our atmosphere was non-traditional.)

Funeral Home "Humor"

THERE WERE ALSO THE JOKES, WHICH I GOT MORE OF THAN MY SISTER, given the guys I grew up with. I have only fond memories of all of them. More than half of the fifteen of them are now deceased: "Hey Danks, your old man is the last one to let you down." "Hey Gus (my nickname), everyone's *dying* to get into your house." And on and on. My father used to get a regular diet of this, too. The odd thing about it was that whoever said things like this said it as if we had never heard it before. We had. So no funeral director jokes please. Trust me, your own local funeral directors will greatly appreciate not hearing them, too.

Enlightened Understanding

GROWING UP IN A FUNERAL HOME WITH DEATH TAUGHT ME ABOUT life. And I'm far from the only one. In an excerpt from "Lessons I Learned Growing Up Around a Funeral Home" (in a small California town), Tess Whitehurst says:

"There were many challenging things about my childhood, but I am overwhelmed with gratitude when I think of being raised around death. It's taught me so much about how to live. [...] *I really can't think of a better place to grow up.*

Here's some of what I've learned:

- Everyday moments are the most precious things.
- It's always the things like reading a book to my nephew, or laughing at an inside joke with my partner, or petting my cat that stand out.
- Crying deeply means you're doing something right.
- At the funeral home, all the beauty and tragedy of life comes to the surface and just hangs there in the air. You see plainly that to love is to grieve and to grieve is to love.
- Everyone is dearer than they seem.
- Even when it was obscured by seemingly challenging character flaws, none of the flaws were who they are—only the light was, only the love. That's why to hear someone eulogized, you would think they were the best person who ever lived—because they were! Just like everyone else is."

The funeral home experience provided our family with an enlightened, but certainly not full, understanding of what death means. It would have been virtually impossible for us not to have been affected in some way by our unique geography. We saw many bodies come in, be embalmed and cosmetically prepared for a viewing – "the wake" as some people still call it – move on shortly to a service in the funeral home or church (on many of those occasions at St. Lawrence, I was one of the altar boys), and then to the cemetery, which was the most common procedure when I was growing up in the 1950s.

The Saddest Times

CLOSING THE CASKET AT THE FUNERAL HOME, OR AT A CHURCH, IS ONE of the saddest times. I've found it is far better to have everyone say their last goodbye, and then have the casket closed by the funeral director and his assistant without anyone else in the room. This is the procedure that my father always used.

When the casket is closed in a church, it is often turned from public view or moved off to the side, so that the lining can be fitted inside and the casket locked. It can occasionally cause a real burst of emotion when it's done in full view of everyone. I witnessed it once. It came out of the blue – and it was heart rending. It just emphasizes the finality of it all.

Other sad times are when the final goodbye is given at the funeral home and when family members cover their loved one with the silken blanket, when the casket or urn comes down the aisle leaving a church followed by the family and friends, or when everyone takes leave at the gravesite.

When favorite hymns or songs are played at a service, it can also be very emotional. A particular one, "I Am the Bread of Life," which is familiar to Catholics, reminds me of many funerals I've been to. It always makes my eyes fill up. I can't even get through singing it anymore. It just shows that even though the worst may have passed, some of the emotion of that day, and from the past, is still there, lying just below the surface.

When someone dies, it almost seems unreal, but at these moments the realism of it has always hit me. Fortunately, things often start to gradually improve after the goodbyes are finished. It's a great example of resilience, something that's important in everyday life, too.

Cemeteries, Cremations, and Body Donations to Science

TODAY, CREMATION HAS BECOME A FAR MORE COMMON ALTERNATIVE – now probably the option in more than half of all funerals. (There may be some regional variation in this.) At least part of this was due to the Catholic Church's removal of the general prohibition against cremation. It is also due primarily to the fact that having the deceased cremated is less expensive than having a traditional funeral with a casket and vault. (It is mandatory in most cemeteries that the casket be placed into a concrete vault to protect it and to minimize the subsidence of the soil over top of it. You'll notice in many older cemeteries that this was not done, with the undulating landscape being a dead giveaway.)

Whether to have a burial or cremation is an individual and family choice. I like being able to visit a cemetery, knowing that a loved one's body is there. It helps make the person's memory come more alive for me. Others might say, "It's all in your head," my father probably included; because you can recall a loved one if they have been cremated just the same.

Another alternative is to have the deceased's body donated to benefit medical science. This typically would be something that the deceased indicated they wanted. Local medical universities can provide details on this option, which can also dramatically reduce the cost of final expenses.

Taking Security Precautions at Home

IT'S HARD FOR ANY RESPECTABLE PERSON TO IMAGINE THIS COULD BE true, but there are those who read obituaries to find out what time the funeral service is going to be, presuming that the family home will be empty then, who take this opportunity to burglarize the premises. New York police apprehended a woman who made a habit of doing this. The same article mentioned cases in Massachusetts, Illinois, and Indiana, so they're not isolated incidents.

Ask friends or neighbors to keep a watch on your home and advise the police that you will be attending a family funeral. Be sure to lock all your windows and doors and put on the burglar alarm if you have one. Alternatively, it can be useful if a few friends stay in the property, or at least outside, to give things an occupied look.

Cemetery Observations

IT'S A REFLECTIVE EXPERIENCE TO WALK THROUGH A CEMETERY. I'VE done it many times. The quotations on some older tombstones and their artistry are really something. Stone carvers, and sometimes ships' carvers, carved them. I've seen some touching things. It brought tears to my eyes when I walked through the cemetery in Marblehead, Massachusetts that's up on a hill looking out to the sea. I saw a little marker for a young baby who died in the 1700s. I visualized the young parents at the baby's gravesite so long ago. Of the thousands of grave markers we see, at one time virtually all of them had an assemblage of family members and friends standing there for the final farewell.

I visited my parents' graves recently. It struck me that I couldn't remember standing there when they were having their last gathering, thirty years ago for my mother and seventeen years ago for my father. The memory gets fuzzy after a while, although they are still missed, just like your loved ones are.

In the material world, that's what it all comes down to. It's one hell of a lesson in life. No matter who you were or how powerful you were, or weren't, it all ends at that small piece of earth. It's humbling. Something we should remember in dealing with people in our daily lives. It's similar to when "the big boss" may have been revered, or perhaps feared, when she/he was in control. But after they retire, any glow that was on the rose may come off quickly, especially if they haven't treated others well during their tenure. It's that in spades once we see someone's burial site or know that they've been cremated.

Grave Matters

IT'S TOUCHING TO SEE THE LOVE SHOWN BY THE FLOWERS AND remembrances people put on the graves of their loved ones, especially on certain commemorative and holiday occasions. I believe that it gives families comfort. I have never done it though. My father was very explicit about it: "DON'T put anything on my grave!" So even though I visit my parents' graves, I've never left anything there, except my prayers and thanks for all they did for us, including the struggles to pay for our college educations.

My parents have modest rectangular markers with their names, birth and death year, and a quotation. My father is on the left. His reads, "This is the day the Lord has made." My mother's on the right says, "Do something beautiful for God." So it's inspiring to read them straight across: "This is the day the Lord has made. Do something beautiful for God." Directions for us – even from the grave. These join many other instructive and educational monuments I've read that provide encouragements, and even humor, sometimes.

Some very old markers reflect philosophical and religious beliefs of the time. Others have very dire warnings for the living, complete with reminders of one's eventual death, including skulls and crossbones, skeletons, a deathly finger pointing upward, and an urn and willow – a traditional symbol of mourning. A very famous admonition was:

Remember me as you pass by,
As you are now, so once was I,
As I am now, so you will be,
Prepare for death and follow me.

I've seen this one many times. It's a strange, but arresting feeling, when it seems as if someone is speaking to you from the grave.

Many of the gravestones in colonial cemeteries are classics that are truly book and photo worthy. The second most visited cemetery in the country, after Arlington National Cemetery in Virginia, is the Granary Burial Ground in Boston. It's down the street from the Boston Common and the Massachusetts State House.

The day I visited there I met the cemetery superintendent who offered to give me a tour. He asked the right guy. The cemetery is fairly small, but its monuments are a mastery of the arts and a lesson in history. It's the final resting places for many famous people, including Samuel Adams, John Hancock, and Paul Revere. Ben Franklin's parents are buried there too. But their son Ben is buried in his adopted city of Philadelphia.

What have I learned
Where'er I've been
From all I've heard, from all I've seen?
What know I more worth the knowing?
What have I done that's worth doing?
What have I sought that I should shun?
What duties have I left undone?"

– Pythagoras

PART III

The Takeaway from Seven Decades

*I've learned things from this specialized experience
in my youth and in the decades since.*

Life Can Be Fragile

I'VE SEEN HEALTHY PEOPLE REDUCED TO DYING IN A RELATIVELY SHORT time, sometimes in an instant. A grade school classmate died a few years after graduating from high school when his car was hit by a train. Another grade school classmate died from an auto accident coming home at night after he had just started college. We had both funerals. Just about anyone today could augment that by recalling young people who died of drug overdoses, something that was rare when I was growing up, but with the opioid crisis today has become all too common. A member of our family died from one.

There are certain things that happen to us in life that aren't preventable, but many times, we do have control and should exercise good judgment so we don't wind up dying ahead of our time because of drug abuse, alcoholism, drinking and driving, smoking, failing to get medical screenings, failing to take prescribed drugs, taking imprudent risks, or by not calling 911 first in any health emergency, instead of calling for advice or driving to the hospital. Life can be somewhat fragile by nature. We shouldn't tempt fate by doing inadvisable things.

The Courage of the Dying

IN ADDITION TO MY MOTHER, I HAVE HAD A FEW FRIENDS WHO DIED from serious illnesses whom I spoke with during their illness. In spite of their having to deal with many unpleasant and painful treatments and many trips to medical facilities, I was impressed by their courage and acceptance of the situation. The same goes for their selfless and loving caregivers. It's probably true that it doesn't do much good to rail against the situation, but to accept things as patiently as they did has been a life lesson for me. I'm sure you know others who have done the same. I hope I can follow the good example they set if I'm ever in the same position. I hope you can too.

Drug Abuse

I'M A FULL-TIME BUSINESS ADMINISTRATION FACULTY MEMBER AT A community college. Each semester I warn my students about the dangers of drug abuse and when someone dies from an accidental overdose, they wind up just as dead. I also tell them that it isn't just speculation on my part because I've seen some of the bodies that resulted from these bad decisions. Aside from being illegal, dealing with drug dealers is also far from the comparative safety of obtaining prescribed drugs from a local pharmacy.

The advent of fentanyl and other powerful drugs like carfentanyl has made the risk all the more dangerous. Carfentanyl is one hundred times stronger than fentanyl and five thousand times more potent than heroin. It is used to anesthetize six-thousand-pound elephants. There's little wonder that the ignorance of drug dealers and the foolish risks users take, kill people.

No high is worth dying for. It's infinitely better to get high on life instead. No drug can fill a hole in someone's soul. The risk takers aren't just younger people, but those in middle age and older. Anyone who needs help should get it, not only in their own interest, but in that of those who love them. I have seen parents standing at the casket of their children who died from an overdose. Words can't describe the sadness.

Giving the Ego a Rest

TO SEE THE WAY SOME PEOPLE ACT, YOU'D BELIEVE THEY THINK THEY'RE indispensable or immortal and that the world couldn't possibly get along without them. A frequent expression of my father's: "We're all useful, but we're not necessary."

None of it lasts. Titles, impressive offices, money, cars, expensive boats, homes, designer fashions, jewelry and well-stocked wine cellars. All these things can be good in themselves. *The question is where is the focus going? Are such things a nice adjunct to life – or life itself?* Other than perhaps a few mementos like photos, a rosary, an Eagles jersey or Yankees cap, or a few trinkets, none of it can come with us when we leave. *The only real thing we can take with us when we go is the good we've done and the reputation we established by helping others.*

A friend and colleague told me that she saw a forerunner of this when she visited an elite nursing home, one where there were no Medicare residents, just all cash-paying customers. She said it hit her that in their former lives they had the best of everything, but now she saw them in their wheelchairs with just a blanket or rosary beads. Sometimes we can't take it with us – even when we're still living. This is a stark reminder to focus on what's really important in life, not on material things or on ourselves.

It's also foolish to spend a life thinking that it's all about us. It isn't. Thinking about it often doesn't make it so. In a material and self-absorbed society, it's easy to center on ourselves and on our own egos. Roman emperor Marcus Aurelius in his still highly relevant guide for life that I'm very fond of, *Meditations*, furnishes us with a vivid perspective on the folly of self-absorbed acquisition and of manufactured self-importance:

"All things fade into the storied past, and in a little while are shrouded in oblivion. Even to men whose lives were a blaze of glory this comes to pass; as to the rest, the breath is hardly out of them before, in Homer's words: "they are lost to sight and hearsay alike."

That's something that's always given me pause.

Hospice Care

WHEN SOMEONE IS TERMINALLY ILL, THERE IS NO NEED TO FACE IT alone. It is a difficult road for the person who is dying and also for the caregivers. There may be a reluctance to ask for this type of assistance for a number of reasons, but the general wisdom is that hospice care should be sought sooner than it typically is.

Sometimes the person who is ill may not want it, feeling that they are being pushed aside or that they don't want to have their privacy invaded. The practical matter though is that it can be colossally hard on caregivers to do all that is needed, both physically and psychologically. That is something that might have to be tactfully pointed out to the person who is ill.

Other times it may be the caregiver who does not want to ask for help because they want to do it themselves, feeling that they might be shirking their responsibilities if they don't or that they might be hastening the patient's death by doing so. But the benefits of hospice can make things far better for both the patient and the caregiver. The patient's health should not be the only consideration, either. The health of caregivers needs to be considered too, not only in their own interest, but in the interest of the patient. In many situations, if the caregiver goes down, the consequences for many patients would be substantial.

Hospice care can be offered in a patient's home, that of a family member or friend, in a hospital, a hospice center, or in a nursing facility or assisted-living setting.

As Dr. Atul Gawande pointed out earlier in his book, *Being Mortal*, engaging hospice sooner not only brings about a better quality of life for the patient, it often helps to extend life too.

The excellent article, "Why Hospice Care Could Benefit Your Loved One Sooner Than You Think." (*Nation* 1/29/2015) refers to hospice as a valuable, often overlooked, and generous benefit from

Medicare for those caring for a family member or friend. It provides excellent detail and advice on the benefits of hospice for all concerned. Coverage is also provided by private insurance carriers and the Veterans Administration.

"Medicare has paid for most hospice care received in the United States. Beneficiaries are eligible for hospice care when they are entitled to Medicare Part A and are certified by a physician as having a life expectancy of six months or less if the illness runs its normal course. However, living longer than six months doesn't mean the patient loses the benefit. After the initial certification period, each beneficiary receives an unlimited number of additional 60-day periods.

People often wait too long before seeking hospice care. In the United States, the average length of hospice care is less than 60 days with 30 percent of those who elect hospice care dying in seven days or fewer. It seems that misinformation about the benefit coupled with our general discomfort talking about end of life prevents Medicare beneficiaries and their family from taking advantage of the valuable benefit.

Hospice care provides many services through health and social service professionals joined by volunteers:

– Comfort care
– Maintenance care for existing chronic conditions
– Emotional, social, psychological and spiritual support
– Needed drugs, medical supplies and equipment
– Mentoring individuals, family, and friends on best practices in patient care
– Services like speech and physical therapy, which can be accessed when needed
– If receiving hospice at home, payment for short-term inpatient care is available when symptoms become too much to manage or when caregivers need a respite break to take care of themselves
– Grief counseling is available

Those receiving care are allowed to keep their regular physician or nurse practitioner to oversee their care or to receive care from the doctor associated with the hospice organization."

Final Wishes of the Deceased

THE DECEASED CAN'T SPEAK FOR THEMSELVES ONCE THEY HAVE GONE ahead. But out of respect, they're entitled to the type of funeral they wanted. To ensure that, it's important to ask those questions, ideally when the person is still in good health, but certainly when it appears that death is reasonably imminent or when someone is in hospice care. This isn't something most family members want to bring up, but it's important to do it, so that after someone has passed there isn't a guessing game about what they wanted or family arguments about it. This is one of the big advantages of people pre-planning their own funerals.

This would include what they would like to wear when they are viewed – and they may or may not want to be. Sometimes a man might say, "Don't put any tie on me! I never wore one." Paul, one of the older guys I grew up with, who was always kind to me, was viewed in a flannel shirt. It was him. It looked perfectly fine. Others would indicate the suit and tie or dress they want to be buried in. A colleague's mother said she wanted her nails to be polished. It's those nice small things we can do for those we care about. Doing things the way they wanted them, can be comforting.

Highly Memorable Funerals

FOR MOST OF US, THE MOST MEMORABLE FUNERALS ARE THOSE involving our own family members and close friends. One of my cousins and his wife lost their daughter after a long battle against a rare disease, just as she became a teenager. They all gave it everything they had. My cousin's fellow Philadelphia police officers held benefits to raise money for their expenses and took turns working his shifts so he wouldn't lose a paycheck. That type of kindness is remarkable and unmatched and can never be forgotten. It never has been.

Their daughter's funeral Mass was as special as it could be. Her eighth grade classmates all came to the funeral. In total, the church had a thousand family members and friends. Our oldest cousin, who was a Monsignor, said her funeral Mass. I know he was very concerned about the remarks he would make in his eulogy, but his kind and gentle words were one of his finest hours.

When we left the church, there were about a dozen police officers from the Philadelphia Police Motorcycle Unit out front, each standing at attention next to their cycles in just an indescribable tribute to my cousin's daughter, her mother and her father. They led the funeral procession out the very busy Roosevelt Boulevard in Philadelphia, using a protocol reserved for dignitaries to block off each cross street, providing for an uninterrupted journey to their daughter's carefully selected and peaceful final resting place. In spite of the great grief my cousin and his wife had over their daughter's long illness and her passing, at the funeral luncheon they went from table to table to speak with everyone and to thank them for coming. Sometimes we can show great strength that we never know we have until we're put into a situation to demonstrate it. The whole day touched me greatly.

Probably my father's largest funeral was one for a family of five – the mother and father and their three children – who all died in a house fire. There were five hearses and a large number of people. Because of the tragic nature of it, it was also covered by the media. In the funeral parlor, my father had three small white caskets in the middle between those of their parents – together in both life and death.

In another tragic event, in Gloucester City, New Jersey there was a house fire. The parents survived the fire, but three of their children died, along with three brave firefighters who perished trying to rescue them, two of them from an adjoining community. Although I didn't know him personally, the youngest firefighter went to the same high school I did. Out of respect, many others and I went to his funeral Mass at St. Mary's Church. The crowd overflowed into the street and was so large that a number of priests came outside to distribute Communion. His brother firefighters lifted his casket on to the fire truck to be borne to his final place of rest. An annual scholarship in his honor is given annually in his high school to honor his memory and his courage.

Something that many probably have not seen is funerals for priests and nuns. Four of my father's sisters were Catholic nuns. The funerals for the religious are different because many of the mourners are primarily fellow sisters and priests who process in together, representing the good and the sacrifices that the deceased stood for. It highlights the nature of their unique societies, much in the same way that there is a brotherhood of military, police officers, and firefighters. The rituals at these ceremonies are special and inspirational.

My cousin, James J. Flood, the Monsignor whom I spoke of earlier, had been an assistant rector at St. Charles Seminary in Philadelphia for twenty-five years and a pastor of Saint Margaret's Parish in Narberth, just outside the city, for about the same period of time. He had a large funeral, which included a procession into the church of over seventy-five priests, a number of whom he had taught in the seminary.

He was a sterling example of caring and kindness to our large family. (My father was one of fourteen children.) Father Jim was the rock who was there for all of us. He was our oldest cousin and the first one to die. A reminder, too, that there now was a passing of generations – and that our own passing would come in turn. He had only been retired for a few years when he was stricken with an illness from which he would not recover. He joined others, whom I mentioned earlier, who faced the end of his life with great courage and set an example for us in death that he set for us in life.

Finding What to Say at
Viewings and Funerals

SOME FIND IT DIFFICULT TO ATTEND VIEWINGS AND FUNERALS BECAUSE they feel as if they don't know what to say. The main thing to remember is that *your mere presence says 90 percent of what needs to be said.* Families appreciate that someone took the time to come, especially when they know the person has come a distance or hasn't seen the deceased for a long time. One of my classmates said, "It's the people that you don't expect to come that can really make things special."

Funerals and viewings used to be occasions when attendees always dressed appropriately. Most people still do. But as in going to nicer restaurants or going to the theater and other venues, dress has become far more informal, sometimes bordering on, or crossing over to, the inappropriate. For funerals, it's a sign of respect for the deceased and the family to stay within proper bounds. I always wear a suit and tie to viewings and funerals. I made an exception recently when I went to a morning service in a funeral home for a former classmate. His obituary clearly stated "casual attire requested". It fit him, great fisherman that he was. I hadn't seen this type of request before, but thought it was a good one. If it's ok with the family, then it seems just fine to me.

When I was in high school, we used to visit my friend Tom's home in Gloucester where we frequently passed the time drinking beer, telling jokes, and fooling around. Sadly, he died at forty-two of a rare disease. And over thirty years later, I'm still here. There is no explaining why his life ended so soon – and why mine and others' didn't. A great deal of light and good humor went out of the world when he died.

Tom's father had a law office in their home and a long-time secretary, Ruth, who tried to work while we were making our usual racket. On more than a few occasions she had to come back to the kitchen to ask us to hold it down. Ruth was as nice as she could be and treated us like friends. When she died, far too young, I went to her viewing. I told the family that I hadn't seen her in decades but wanted them to know how nice she had always been to us. It was something they appreciated. Sometimes, just a small mention of appreciation for something the deceased did or sharing a memory can help.

Just saying that you're sorry is also good, although your presence already says that, so you might not feel the need to verbally express it. My cousin Tom and his wife Sarah, who both suffered painful losses of loved ones, told me that saying, "I'm sorry for your loss. I know that it hurts," serves a double purpose. It expresses sorrow and also shows empathy.

A colleague told me that she says, "I am sorry to hear that he/she passed. I will keep everyone in my prayers." That's something people seem to appreciate. Even though they may not be believers, they recognize the sincerity of the good thoughts.

Be careful of saying things that have sometimes been said, such as "At least he's not suffering anymore," or if it's a child that died, "You can have more children." That may be true, but it won't be the one who has passed.

The same thing applies to elderly parents. Some people don't get it when they make comments like, "Well, she was ninety." That may be true, *but she was still their mother,* no matter how old she was when she died. In any case, it can be upsetting for family members to hear insensitive comments at times like this.

Keep it simple. Sometimes the person you're speaking with will want to talk. Other times, the line behind you and the person's own feelings at the time, may prevent that. The important thing is that you came. If you are on the fence about going, go. It will help.

If you're in the receiving line yourself, don't presume that everyone you thought would come to the viewing or service will do so. Families are far more likely to remember who did not come when they were expected, than those who did. It's better not to judge.

There may have been reasons why someone couldn't come. It's also possible they didn't know that your loved one died. Sometimes I haven't found out about someone's death until months afterward, even those I had been close with – and I read the obituaries every day.

One thing that can help you find something to say when you get your turn to speak to family members is to look carefully at all the photos or the video that many families have at viewings. It is a very instructive experience. It shows truly valued occasions. Following them sequentially provides a window into someone's life. It is especially useful if you have many blanks to fill in because you haven't seen the deceased for quite a while.

I went to the funeral Mass of one of my high school classmates recently. I hadn't seen him since we graduated fifty-five years ago. I saw photos of him as a baby, his wedding, his children, grandchildren, backyard picnics, shore and boat outings, vacation photos and many of him and his wife. What a privilege. It can give a family a real lift by paying your respects, whether you just go in to call before the service or stay for it. I recommend it as a small thing we can do for those who can use support at a sad time.

Sometimes the tables are turned. Joe McCullough, who was an attorney, died suddenly of a heart attack early Easter morning over twenty years ago. He was an exemplary man and a good friend to me. I managed his campaign for Congress over forty years ago. He helped many people during his lifetime. Joe had one of the longest viewing lines I've ever seen. Someone remarked, "Who would ever believe that this was a line for a lawyer's funeral?" Lawyers get many jokes about them too, just like funeral directors.

Everyone admired Joe and was willing to wait for two hours to pay their respects. He and his wife Joan had four children and adopted two others. They were models of charity in many respects. People came to offer consolation to his widow. But in spite of the suddenness of her husband's death, she was cheering up the mourners. He was too much. So was she.

We often hear things around the time of someone's death that can be uplifting. Around the time of Joe's passing, which was a real shock to me, I remember someone saying that the happiest birth-day we will ever have is the first one we spend with the Lord. While I know some don't share that belief, Joe and Joan were certainly people who did.

Similarly, the anniversary of one's death, and the first of every-thing: the first month anniversary, the first Thanksgiving, the first Christmas, and the deceased's birthday, are often sad reminders. Although often thought of sadly, some have described the date of death as the day someone went to Heaven. Some may see this as trying to put a good spin on a sad matter, but if we give it some thought, we may be able to find other similar positives to get us through a difficult time.

Eulogies Can Be Excellent Teachers

HAVE YOU EVER HEARD ANYONE IN A EULOGY, GOING ON AND ON, about how much money someone had, how many homes they had or how beautiful their outfits and jewelry were? What gets emphasized is what counts: the kind of a mother or father the deceased was, how he was a friend that helped those in need, how she took care of her parents or siblings, how they were ready to lend a hand to anyone and to their community, how they inspired others, the humorous stories and phrases that were them, and *how the person made a real difference* in the lives of others.

Not everyone wants a eulogy. A friend said her father-in-law didn't want his past life told at the funeral. He said, "Bury me. I lived my life, go live yours." Excellent advice for everyone, especially for those who mourn to the point that they don't live their lives in a full way.

I attended a funeral lunch where several men stood up and said how the quiet, unassuming, and humble man, who had just been buried in a local cemetery had made such a difference in their lives, some of them being turned completely around to march in a new and far better direction. What a wonderful legacy to leave.

A ninety-five-year-old physician, the father of one of my classmates, and beloved by his family, died recently. He was a model man having served in the US Navy and, for many decades, as a community and industrial physician, football team doctor, and caring health provider to many nuns and priests. A number of my classmates, now in their seventies, had him for their childhood physician.

His oldest grandson gave him a wonderful tribute: "We treasured the times we learned from him. He reminded me of a Norman Rockwell painting. He was good, holy, and honorable." It would be good to hear such comments about ourselves. He concluded by saying, "The legacy of those who pass is in our hands now." And so it is for all of us.

To emulate the good, exceptional men and women have done, is quite a charge. We might not be able to imitate it or to match it. The important thing is that we are our best selves.

As I was driving away from the church, many of those attending the doctor's service were standing outside. I drove past a man crossing the street holding the hands of what appeared to be his two small grandchildren. I heard him say, "He must have known a lot of people." He did. And he was good to all of them. That's why so many came to pay their respects. Those in their nineties typically have very small turnouts for fairly obvious reasons. This was a striking exception – and everyone knew why.

Eulogies serve as measures of goodness and can be real learning experiences for the living. I find them instructive in terms of how a life has been well lived and how the deceased gained the love and respect of those who knew her/him. They often provide substantive food for thought for us to consider in modeling our own lives.

Stephen Covey in his New York Times best seller, *The Seven Habits of Highly Effective People,* suggests that we should write our own eulogy – what we would want speakers to say about us after we're gone. Then use those thoughts as a guide for our own life. It would surely produce many improved eulogies in the future.

The Funeral Meal

AFTER THE SERVICE HAS CONCLUDED, EITHER AT A HOUSE OF WORSHIP, a funeral home, or a graveside service, it is often customary to invite the attendees for lunch at a local restaurant or other facility, such as a church hall or a fire house. Sometimes everyone returns to the family home or to a relative's. I suggest doing it at an outside facility. It brings a punctuated end to the day's events. When it's in a home, people can linger beyond the time that the family might like. Days like this are difficult and tiring enough without unnecessarily extending them.

A funeral meal is an extension of hospitality and a nice courtesy for those who came to the funeral. Whether to go or not is an individual decision. Obviously, immediate family would go. Others just need to decide whether they are going to feel comfortable going. Sometimes a family member may directly ask you to come. Unless there is some reason why you can't, it's good to accept the invitation.

If at all possible, hold the funeral meal in a location proximate to the last place everyone gathered, to eliminate unnecessary driving. One of my readers said she had a morning viewing and Mass in the church for both her parents' funerals, followed by a luncheon downstairs in the church. This would especially work well if a burial is going to be private or if there already has been a cremation. The same procedure was followed for my cousin, Monsignor Flood. It is useful to follow this protocol too when the interment is going to take place the same day, but when the cemetery is at a distance and most people wouldn't be coming to the interment.

A funeral luncheon for fifty to a hundred people can be a real expense. If there is a suspicion that the cost may be a burden for the family, it's nice for those with resources to offer financial assistance. An overture like this should be made in private and tactfully. Speaking with the funeral director about it first might be a way to get some insight about what would be appropriate and how it might be handled, even anonymously, as they probably have handled similar situations before. The same overture can be made if there is a thought that there may be a need for assistance with the funeral bill.

Another approach, if the meal is held in a home or hall, is to have people bring what's necessary for the lunch. I went to a subsequent memorial remembrance in a fire hall for a colleague that worked this way and it was lovely. While I don't believe this type of funeral meal is generally common in our area, it is not uncommon in some areas of the country, especially when a church community may take the lead. Sometimes even wedding receptions are held this way.

Occasionally, you may hear some criticism of the fact that about an hour ago, mourners were by a graveside and now they're in a room eating and laughing, and maybe drinking too, and getting back to normal. It can be a positive thing. It helps many families begin the healing process and also gives them a better opportunity to renew relationships and to thank those who came. It's probably also something that the deceased would want to see happening – with their family and friends having a good time together on their account. Sometimes the deceased may have also provided explicit instructions about the kind of get-together they wanted, or what they didn't want.

It's an unfortunate fact of life that in many families, weddings and funerals are some of the rare occasions that family members get to see one another. Funerals especially, as family members get older. But at least it's a touch point. It's a good time to plan for everyone to get together sometime in the future for a happier occasion.

One of our dedicated cousins, Mary Jane, continued the tradition of a Danks Family Reunion every two years at a well-known restaurant at Harborplace in Baltimore. We don't say, "The only time we see everybody is at funerals," as much anymore. It's a good thing for families to plan. We've all been indebted to her and her husband Tom for doing this to help keep our family together.

After Things Are Over,
It Can Get Awfully Lonely

THAT'S WHERE YOU CAN COME IN. FUNERALS ARE A TIME WHEN extensive energy is extended in support of survivors, but it's like a lightning bolt – powerful, but very short. Survivors get support for three days or a week, dropping off sharply after that. It's a hard thing to deal with and can exacerbate feelings of loneliness.

Sometimes family and friends are afraid to approach someone because they feel as if it may be too soon or because "I don't know what to say" or "I don't want to say the wrong thing." *Take the risk and reach out.* You'll be able to sense whether someone wants to talk on the phone, in person, take a walk or go to lunch after you speak with them. Just follow their lead.

If you are one of the survivors, know that people might be reluctant to contact you. *When you're ready, take the lead yourself. Ask them to stop over, take a walk or whatever you would feel good about. Break the ice.* Let others know that you're ready for contact and it will come to you. The worst thing is grieving alone, without support and companionship, when it might be dearly wished for.

If you sense that someone is not ready for contact, just keep it brief and let them know that you are there for them. Instead of the usual, "If there is anything I can do..." suggest a few possibilities. My friend Carla suggested that one thing that can be helpful at the time you first learn of someone's passing is to offer to call people for the family to tell them about the person's death, the funeral arrangements, or to provide other details. It can be a monumental job having to call many relatives and friends, especially when the family may be in shock or grieving, and also perhaps when they wouldn't want to get involved in extended conversations.

Another way to help is to step up to the plate if you see there is something obvious you can do. My cousin Tom, who is now eighty years old, lost his father when he was nine years old. I was too young to know his father, but I know my father admired Uncle Jim very much. He respected him as a man of great character and intellect. He was married to my eldest aunt, Aunt Mary Ellen. Together they created a loving home – and a very clean one too – for their two sons. When she died, my cousin quipped that, "Heaven will be a cleaner place."

When Tom's father died, my grandfather, my father, and his three brothers John, Bill and Joe all stepped in to provide support and guidance to my cousin and to his older brother, who became the Monsignor I mentioned earlier. His parish priests and the Christian Brothers, who were his teachers, provided further guidance. It surely helped them both in a time of need.

E-mailing or texting occasionally can provide support that is only mildly intrusive. One thing that is a dying art is writing a letter or a note of condolence. In today's electronic society, we see far fewer of them than in the past, but they can give someone a real lift.

Putting Your Foot in Your Mouth

OCCASIONALLY, WE MAY INADVERTENTLY PUT OUR FOOT IN OUR mouth. On a few occasions, I asked people, very cheerily, how their summer had been, only to learn that they had lost a close family member that I hadn't heard about. I apologized sincerely, but the damage had been done. Sometimes we don't stay plugged into life the way we should. If we were better at it, we'd be more likely to avoid situations like this.

Even offhanded remarks can potentially cause discomfort. For example, someone can start going off on drug abusers, forgetting, or just learning on the spot, that the person in their company may have lost someone in their family to an overdose.

A colleague told me that it's good to remember that dying due to drug use sometimes starts from an addiction begun after surgery or an accident, when a doctor legitimately prescribed pain killers. Addiction is also a disease, not something that just willpower alone can typically overcome. She also said it's never a good idea just to try a drug once, for fun, because this act can lead to addiction and possibly later death.

Spontaneous utterances just slip out. It's a matter of thinking before we speak – something I should have been far better at during my life. Again, a sincere apology is in order when we realize we inadvertently said something that could cause hurt.

My wife told me that she has had occasions when someone she was speaking with brought up death, after her former husband, and subsequently her son, died. Most of the time, the person making the remark realizes that something they said would have been better left unsaid. It just takes some forethought and judiciousness to avoid circumstances like these.

Handling Grief and Loss

A GOOD FRIEND LOST HIS WIFE OF OVER FORTY YEARS SUDDENLY DUE to a health-related condition. They were very close, had a wonderful family, and had traveled the world together. He told me he had great difficulty dealing with her loss. A friend suggested that he speak to a wise advisor in another city. He spent quite a while with him. He was asked, "How many times do you think a husband and wife die on the same day?" My friend said that it wasn't likely to be very often. The advisor reminded him that in life it is almost uniformly the case that one person dies before the other. He asked him, if he had died first, would he have wanted his wife to be unhappy? He was then able to recognize that his wife would not want him to be unhappy in life either. From that point on, his healing began. The greatest gift we can give to a deceased loved one is a life well and fully lived. It doesn't mean forgetting. It just means adapting for everyone's benefit.

Grief Counseling

A GRIEF SUPPORT GROUP CAN BE HELPFUL, BECAUSE YOU WOULD BE interacting with others who have already gone through the experience. It provides living proof that you can get to a better place, once you've moved farther down the track.

My classmate Trish has been a facilitator of a grief counseling group for over twenty years. She lost her wonderful husband a few years ago. Bob was a terrific guy who was kind to me at times when I needed it. He is also someone whom I spoke of before who endured a great deal with his illness before he died, but never complained once about it – to me or to his wife, and probably not to anyone else either. I spoke with her about grief counseling. She offered these thoughts:

- Grief is unique to everyone. There is no right way or wrong way to grieve.
- Give yourself three or four months after someone's loss to just be. Before that, for most, it's too early to get started with grief support groups.
- One of the best things about being in a grief support group is that you will be with others who understand, but who are not emotionally involved with your loss like family members would be.
- Grieve the way that you want. Don't compare yourself to anyone else.
- You can get paralyzed – just know that you aren't going crazy if you do, for example, you can't think, you can't read, or you can't get anything done.
- Pick realistic goals: "I'm going to get it together and attack all the paperwork on the dining room table for 15 minutes. Then I'm finished." You'll probably wind up finishing more than you thought, but you won't overwhelm yourself by setting unrealistic goals.
- Do what you want to do. Don't be pushed by family, friends, or

anybody else. Sometimes those, often without much prior experience with grief, might say after a while that you should get over it. Remember, that's for you to decide, not them. Everyone grieves differently and at his/her own rate.

- In her role as being a facilitator, she said that spending two hours per week over twelve weeks with those in the group, she saw great growth, from crying often at the start and having trouble talking about their loved one's passing, to where they opened up in a few weeks and started talking about it. A key she says is to "Listen. Listen. Listen. Love. Love. Love – and share."

- It's important to have goals that are important to you – no matter how modest they are.

- It can be difficult for the person who is ill, and also for those grieving afterward, to maintain self-esteem. This situation is no one's fault, but it can be very hard to be your usual, resilient self under these circumstances. Her support group used affirmations to help restore self-esteem to where it should be.

- Over time, people discover that good can come, even from these sad situations. As she said, "Even dragons can bring us gifts. We just have to keep our eyes open for them." In spite of the fact that it was pretty clear after a while that her husband was not going to survive, she said the care giving she was able to provide was a gift of special time together for them. She said, "We had a beautiful time," one she said they may not have had under normal circumstances.

Grief counseling can also be offered on an individual basis from a professional counselor. Those who are having difficulty moving ahead after someone's death should certainly consider it. There is no right or wrong about this. It isn't for everyone. A number of funeral homes have a grief counselor on staff or can recommend one to you. Your physician can do the same.

In the final analysis, while we may get help dealing with grief, we have to gradually pull ourselves back into the realm of normality. English philosopher George Henry Lewes offers an important key, "The only cure for grief is action."

Thinking We Understand Death

THIS CLEARLY TAKES PERSONAL EXPERIENCE. FOR A LONG TIME, because of where I grew up, I thought I had a pretty good handle on death and dying. Because of my atypical upbringing, compared to most people, I probably do. *But there is no understanding that can take the place of actually having a loss of one of your own loved ones.* That was brought home to me when my mother died of breast cancer at seventy-two.

My mother had regular gynecological and breast examinations every six months, and she still died from breast cancer. I know she would want me to tell anyone to get regular checkups. The chances for survival are much better today than they were in 1988 when she died, but fate shouldn't be tempted by skipping appointments or being afraid that they might find something. Is it better to stay away, truly ensuring that they won't be able to find anything? That makes no sense at all. Better to be a little scared and upset than finding out that you waited too long to give anyone the chance to save you.

I had a recurrence of the same feelings when my father died at eighty-six in 2001. I had seen many funerals, viewings and interments already. None was the same as those for my parents. How much more magnified is it for those who bury their spouses and partners, children and close friends, who by society's standards, may have died ahead of their time?

Burying one's own children violates the natural order of things. As a father said to me as he stood in front of his middle-aged son's casket, "It should be me there." It is hard to lose our parents, but if they have lived to a reasonable age, it is something to be expected. Marianne and I were very fortunate to have the parents we had, and to have had them for as long as we did. Many others sadly lost their parents far sooner.

Losing younger children, especially those who have not had the opportunity to experience the many passages of life: a graduation, weddings, having children, and so on, is altogether different. Losing a child, at any age, is difficult.

My grandmother, Nanny, who lived in the funeral home with us for the last ten years of her life, lost her son, my mother's older brother, when she was in her late eighties. He was in his late fifties. I remember seeing how upset she was. He wasn't young like other examples I cited, but one thing hadn't changed in all those years. He was her son. That will affect us at any age.

Marianne said she remembered Nanny just standing by his casket in silence. Then she said, quoting the book of Job, "The Lord giveth and the Lord taketh away. Blessed be the name of the Lord." Marianne said, "The impact of that prayer did not hit me until I had children of my own. Nanny was a woman of great faith." At times like these, faith can be a true help, but it can be hard to come by at times of great loss – even sometimes for people who usually have it.

President Calvin Coolidge, whom I portrayed a few times in a one-man show, lost his son Calvin at the age of sixteen while he served in the White House. Florence Harding, the widow of Warren G. Harding, whom Coolidge replaced when Harding died in office, sent condolences to the Coolidges and said, "No matter how many loving hands may be stretched out, some paths must be tread alone." Loss of a loved one to death is surely one of them, even when we have support.

My cousin, who lost his father at nine, lost a young son at the age of two and a half. He said it was the saddest day of his life. However, he said, looking back on it, "His son's death instituted a chain of events that were unimagined by me at the time." Ultimately, it helped him meet his current wife of many years, have a reconciliation with his former spouse that benefitted his entire family, and have many grandchildren and great-grandchildren that added to their lives.

As colossally unexpected as it might seem, sad events can sometimes yield the seeds for goodness. They can be virtually impossible to see during a time of deep grief and mourning, but it often becomes manifest later on. It's a good reminder that it's often best in life to take the long view.

Some good that can also come from the passing of exemplary people is to do some of the good they could have done, in their memory.

My Classmates' Deaths

I'M GETTING TO A POINT NOW WHERE I AM LOSING FRIENDS AND classmates too regularly. I had a great high school experience at Gloucester Catholic High School in New Jersey, just across the Walt Whitman Bridge from South Philadelphia. If you ever cross that bridge going into New Jersey, look out to the right and you will see a large red brick building that stands out. That was it. Our "Boy's Building" – the palace of fun and good times. Actual learning took place sometimes there, too.

It must have worked fairly well, because many of my classmates have enjoyed great success in their lives: a priest who was the executive vice-president of a major university, two nuns, a major corporate CEO, two judges, a surgeon, a pharmacist, a veterinarian, a human resources manager, two building contractors, an account-ant, excellent administrative assistants and secretaries, many teachers, several communications workers, several career postal workers, two journalists, engineers – including a pioneer female aerospace engineer, an Emmy award winner, an internationally recognized environmental scientist, and several writers and entrepreneurs – just to name a few.

We went a long time with a fairly small number of classmate deaths. We had our fiftieth class reunion six years ago. Three classmates died in a nine-month period right before it. About twenty classmates, out of our class of about one hundred and twenty, have gone ahead so far.

In what I thought an ironic twist of fate, Lew, one of our class-mates, had a Mass said for our late classmates. Since it was on a weekday, many weren't able to attend. Only one other classmate and I saw him read the names of our deceased from the altar. He had some illness himself about the same time. He died not long afterward.

Talk about a model man. After his military service, he spent his life helping young people as a high school history teacher. He never married, but raised two young family members himself, basically because of the kind of person he was. He didn't see it as someone else's job, but as his.

Previously, we gathered about eight guys together for lunch when a classmate was back in New Jersey from Oregon for his mother's funeral. The food came and everyone was ready to dig in. But Lew said "We have to say grace." And he said it – far better than any of the rest of us could. He also used to hand out small cards with a multi-colored "God bless you!" on it. He wasn't even close to what people might sometimes call a "holy roller". It was simply natural to him as the good man he was.

All this brought home several important points to me:

- Live life to the fullest every day.
- Do good in your own way whenever you can. Sometimes you will be the one uniquely suited to do it – and sometimes no one else will do it.
- If people my age are going ahead, I should realize that my number could be called sometime in the not too distant future – and that I might not get much advance notice either. No matter what age we are, none of us may.

Dying Before Their Time

MY FATHER SPENT YEARS IN THE FUNERAL BUSINESS, AS AN APPRENTICE working at other funeral homes and operating his own funeral home for over thirty years, so he saw death up close and personal for a long time. My sister and I were comparatively short-term witnesses. When someone young died, either a child, younger person, or someone middle-aged, I would often say that they died ahead of their time. My father would simply say, "It *was* their time." He wasn't saying that to be heartless. He was a caring and thoughtful person, but had seen so much of it; he knew the truth of it. While funeral directors try to remain objective and clear-headed for the benefit of those they serve, there are occasions when they can't help to be touched by what they see. This certainly is the case for me now. Almost anyone can see the sadness in these premature deaths.

And I can surely understand how a family suffering a grievous loss can find it difficult, if not impossible, to realize, in the shorter term at least, how this is just something that happens in life. It can seem unfair. The same may go for God, too. Sometimes there is just no making sense of it. It seems fruitless to try. There are some things we may get to understand later in life. But there are other things we will never understand.

For those who have faith, it can help to believe that when something happened, it happened for a reason, as unfathomable as it might seem to us. My mother speculated that perhaps someone being taken ahead of their time may have prevented something much worse that could have happened later. We see daily occurrences of these sad things in the news, too. In line with this, it would be wise not to say to anyone grieving that, "It was God's will." They may process things that way eventually, but funerals aren't the time to bring it up.

As you might expect, when someone doesn't die when it's clearly expected, as in the classic case of a one-hundred-and-one-year-old man pulled a week later from the rubble of a Nepal earthquake, it can make us wonder why. I thought of my father immediately. It wasn't that man's time.

In a similar vein, I've been to funerals where someone very old and feeble walks down the aisle. It's hard not to think, "There's a good chance he's going to be next." Then two weeks later, you'll hear about some other family member or friend who died unexpectedly in their forties.

We're All Going to Get Some Surprises

I DROVE MY FATHER TO ONE OF HIS YOUNGER SISTER'S FUNERALS outside Philadelphia. She had been a Sister of St. Joseph for over fifty years, joining three of his other sisters who pre-deceased her, who also had over fifty years service as Catholic nuns. Since my father was then the oldest surviving sibling, I couldn't help but think sitting next to him that his time might not be far away. It wasn't. He died three weeks later with a heart attack, while planting a small tree in his side yard after lunch. It was a blessing that at his sister's funeral meal, he saw many members of his family that he would not have seen otherwise.

After his heart attack, he spent the next four days in the hospital on life support. The neurologist said that he would not recover. Following my father's often expressed wish that no extraordinary means should be taken, my sister and I agreed to have him removed from life support. He died with each of us holding his hand, one on each side. When it became clear that he was not going to recover, it seemed selfish to keep him here by artificial means. From our perspective, it was also keeping him from going to Heaven.

After his life support was removed, his breathing became labored. Marianne said, "I think he stopped breathing," and I agreed. Then something truly amazing happened. We both thought my father had died, because there was no breathing at all, and he was perfectly still for what seemed at least like a minute. Suddenly, he opened his eyes and he stared straight ahead – but not at either of us. He had a big smile on his face as if he saw something or someone. Then, after about five seconds or so, his face relaxed. I've often speculated that when we go ahead, God, our family and friends will be there to greet us. Seeing this did little to dissuade me from that speculation. Whatever it was, it must have been something good. In spite of being around death for a good part of my life, my father was the only person I have ever seen die.

Honoring Those Who Have Died, but Honoring Yourself Too

ALL OF US ARE ALLOTTED A CERTAIN AMOUNT OF TIME. IT'S PROBABLY good most of the time that we don't know how much time we have left. *But the best thing we can do is to try to honor the person who died by making the most of our own remaining life in memory of theirs, by enjoying our lives, and by trying to do kind and meaningful things.*

It serves no purpose to permanently curl up in grief and not to value and enjoy our lives. They would only want the very best for you, so honor them by making that a purpose of your remaining life.

If the opportunity comes along to remarry or re-couple with a loving partner, take it. You can both have better lives for it. And don't worry about what other people might think. You're the one who may have to go to sleep alone and not have anyone to share evenings and vacations with, not them.

Do whatever makes you happy, just don't settle. Reach out. Someone may be coming toward you. There is no disloyalty to a former spouse or partner in this. They had all the life that was allotted to them. Don't live someone else's life. Live your own. The cold fact is that we are only going to get as much time as we are going to get. Make the most of it.

Some survivors may be content to stay alone. I know people who have lost their partner. I doubt they will ever marry or get into a relationship again. It's a personal choice, but for those who might be open to it, now or later, I offer some thoughts from my e-book, *Dating Advice for Women*, which is in the excerpt that follows. While it was written for women, it applies equally well to men:

LIFE AFTER THE DEATH OF A PARTNER

"Forgetting those things which are behind, and reaching forth unto those things which are before, I press toward the mark." – Philippians 3:13

There's a different kind of hurt when someone loses their love to death. If it's sudden, it's hard to handle emotionally, and sometimes financially. It can also be the result of a long illness, which is draining emotionally and physically.

The length of the survivor's recovery can be affected by many factors including the need for companionship. It can also be affected by who comes into their life in the future.

While a deceased partner may be sorely missed, the problem a survivor may face is loneliness. Some cope by spending more time with family and friends and by taking up new interests. For some, that's enough. New relationships aren't for everyone.

I had a wonderful and perpetually cheerful aunt who was widowed for years. She never remarried. She could have easily. She seemed content and enjoyed spending time with her children and grandchildren. But other women have loneliness and a longing that only having another companion can satisfy. *There's a big difference between being content and contenting yourself.* If what you want is love and companionship, be open to possibilities. In the meantime, be peaceful with your current situation and fill your life with whatever interests you.

There may be a wave of guilt about wanting love again. There shouldn't be. Your deceased spouse or partner received all their allotted time. Hopefully, you shared a good relationship. Keep those memories in that special place in your heart no one can touch. Any caring new love will be respectful enough to help you honor that.

It's hard to imagine that a loving partner wouldn't want you to be happy again. You're still here and deserve to have a life. Value the love you had. Remember the good times always and move ahead. You have to love your own life. You shouldn't let it be controlled by anyone, including the wishes of a loved one that's gone ahead.

I would also not feel bound by, or make, any promises about never getting married again or whom to be buried with. These are often promises made under duress of one form or another. It's unreasonable for a spouse to extract such a promise from a partner, and it's an unwise one to make if there is any possibility you might wish to make a different choice later. Each partner should simply trust the other to do whatever he or she thinks is sensible when the time comes. No one knows what the future holds.

For those with a religious belief, sometimes there is also a concern about, "What happens when I get to Heaven? Who would I be with?" My mother was a wise and charitable person. I asked her that question in my younger days. She said, "People shouldn't worry about things like that. God will have a way to take care of it." That was good enough for me. Irrespective of one's belief system, it's not sensible to worry about things you have no control over.

Make the best use of your time. Make love part of it. You will probably be surprised later to know you could be truly happy again. Some might say, "I could never get married or have a relationship again. There will never be another partner like mine." That's true. There won't be. They were an original. We all are. Seeking another relationship doesn't just mean conducting a search for a clone of a deceased loved one. It means finding a different love with another person with praiseworthy characteristics.

My father was married to my mother for forty-eight years when she died. He married a good, caring woman ten months later. They were both happy for the next thirteen years until my father died at eighty-six. Just because you're in your forties or beyond, don't think that you're through and that having a relationship with a man isn't possible. Don't think about it as the impossible dream. Make the possible one happen. If my father and my stepmother could find happiness in their seventies, there's still a whole lot of hope left for you.

One of my reviewers told me a story about a couple who met in an assisted living facility. They were remarried in their nineties and had four years together. The lady remarked, "Why should I sit here by myself when he could be with me. We're good company for each other." It almost brings tears to your eyes, doesn't it? Talk about keeping hope alive. So please don't think that you must be washed up if you're in your sixties and haven't found someone yet. It's never too late to find happiness.

If you're lonely, give love another chance. If you meet the right person, they will make it easier for you to do it. You may both have memories – good and not so good. Together you can build a future. You're not abandoning your former life and its memories. You're adjusting to a changing situation and creating a new life for yourself.

Don't think your heart only has so much room in it that when someone new comes into it, it has to push someone else out. Think of it as a huge, expandable reservoir that has room for all the love it can hold. As Zelda Fitzgerald said, "Nobody has ever measured, not even poets, how much a heart can hold."

Don't worry what other people think. Sometimes children and friends get upset when a widow decides to date again. They don't have the same perspective because of age or because they haven't been through the same experience. They don't have to live your life, you do. While they are well meaning most of the time, they're not the ones who have to take walks alone, eat alone, spend evenings alone, or go to bed without the warmth and comfort of loving arms around them. Listen to your heart. You *can* be happy again.

Improving Perspective

What follows adds a beautiful and hopeful perspective from Benjamin Franklin, who wrote this letter to offer his condolences to a cousin for a relative who died. Since this was written in colonial times, the language may sound slightly awkward to us, but the message is still clear. If you have lost someone dear to you, I hope you find comfort in it:

To Miss Hubbard

I condole with you. We have lost a dear and valuable relation. But it is the will of God and nature that these mortal bodies be laid aside when the soul is to enter real life. This is rather an embryo state, a preparation for living. A man is not completely born until he be dead. Why then should we grieve that a new child is born among the immortals, a new member added to their happy society?

We are spirits. That bodies should be lent to us while they can afford us pleasure, assist us in acquiring knowledge, or in doing good for our fellow creatures, is a kind and benevolent act of God. When they become unfit for these purposes and afford us pain, instead of an aid become an incumbrance, and answer none of the intentions of which they were given, it is equally kind and benevolent that a way be provided to get rid of them. Death is that way. We ourselves in some cases, prudently choose a partial death. A mangled, painful limb which cannot be restored we willingly cut off. He who plucks out a tooth, parts with it freely, since the pain goes with it, and he who quits the whole body, parts at once with all pains and possibilities of all pains and diseases which it was liable to or capable of making him suffer.

Our friend and we were invited abroad to a party of pleasure which is to last forever. His chair was ready first and he is gone before us. We could not conveniently start together, and why should you and I be grieved at this, since we are soon to follow and know where to find him.

Until Next Time

I'VE WRITTEN EIGHT BOOKS SO FAR. IF YOU'D LIKE TO FIND SOME OTHER topics I've written on, see my other books on Amazon and posts on my LinkedIn page. I hope this book, my other books, and my LinkedIn posts may help you. That's why I wrote them. Best wishes for a long, fulfilling and happy life, and a peaceful passing with few regrets.

Larry Danks
helpfulmedia@yahoo.com

Always have hope:
For oft, when on my couch I lie
In vacant or in pensive mood,
They flash upon that inward eye
Which is the bliss of solitude;
And then my heart with pleasure fills,
And dances with the daffodils.
—From "Daffodils" – William Wordsworth

Focus on what's truly important:
Ten thousand flowers in spring, the moon in autumn,
a cool breeze in summer, snow in winter.
If your mind isn't clouded by unnecessary things,
this is the best season of your life.
—Wu Men

Acknowledgements

Everyone here has experience with happiness – and with loss and grieving, too. Their insights, contributions and support, both past and present, have been an invaluable help to me in writing this book:

My wife Dee, for all her help in reviewing the manuscript multiple times and making helpful content and writing suggestions.

My sister, Chaplain Dr. Marianne Danks, D. Min., Trinity Health Senior Communities.

"My Brother," Jack Marinella.

Mary Kraemer, MD and Co-Director, Temple University Hospital Palliative Care Team, Professor of Medicine, Lewis Katz School of Medicine

My High School Classmates:
Trish Cullen Powell
Tom Heim, Esq.
Kathy Morris Lynch
Jim Orr
Ed Poole MD, FACS
Tom Worrell

My Cousins:
Bill and Pat Danks
Tom and Sarah Flood

Colleagues and Friends:
Maria Aria
Joe Hamill
Dr. Raman Kolluri
Dr. Carla Monticelli

Recommended Self-Help Reading

Authentic Happiness – Martin Seligman
How to identify your signature strengths. Your success comes from trying to incorporate them into your life as much as possible.

Flourish – Martin Seligman
A subsequent development to *Authentic Happiness*, demonstrating that multi-faceted well-being should be the goal in life, not happiness alone.

Fifty Classics Series –Tom Butler-Bowdon
An entire series of "Fifty Classics" on self-help books about success, prosperity, psychology, business, economics, politics, and philosophy. They are eminently readable and provide the essence of many famous works.

Never Too Late To Be Great – Tom Butler-Bowdon
Goals can be set and successes can be achieved, at any age.

The Happiness Curve: Why Life Gets Better After Fifty – Jonathan Rauch
How happiness declines from the optimism of youth, descending into a trough in middle age, and rebounds as we age.

The Positive Shift: Mastering Mindset to Improve Happiness, Health, and Longevity – Catherine Sanderson
Thought patterns exert a substantial influence on our psychological and physical health. How to make minor tweaks in your mindset to help live a longer and happier life.

Happiness and Success Website – Lawrence J. Danks
Contains over one hundred summaries of articles on positive psychology, motivation, inspiration, success, and my own contributions.

Access it through: ccc.webstudy.com
User Name: happiness
Password: success
Click "Timeline" then "Expand All"

Thrive: The Third Metric to Redefining Success and Creating a Life of Well-Being, Wisdom, and Wonder – Arianna Huffington
Dealing with burnout and stress and achieving well-being.

The Power of Habit – Charles Duhigg
How to create positive habits and how to break bad ones.

Being Mortal: Medicine and What Matters in the End – Dr. Atul Gawande
An unexcelled guide to medical care and to end care for those facing terminal illness and for those responsible for them.

Grit – Angela Duckworth
How grit (perseverance) is an elemental component of success.

Too Soon Old, Too Late Smart – Gordon Livingston
Dr. Livingston uses his experience as a practicing psychiatrist to help deal positively with many of life's common problems. Anyone reading this will see themselves in it.

Flow – Mihaly Cziksentmihalyi
The world's leading expert on flow studies explains the concept of flow and how bringing more of it into your life can provide for increased happiness.

Ikigai: The Japanese Secret to a Long and Happy Life – Hector Garcia and Francesc Miralles
How to infuse each day with meaning and find a reason for living as a key to a longer and happier life, including advice from contented ninety- and one-hundred-year-olds.

Peak: Secrets of the New Science of Expertise – Anders Ericsson and Robert Pool
How deliberate practice creates experts and can help others improve to become more successful.

The How of Happiness: A Scientific Approach to Getting The Life You Want – Sonja Lyubomirsky
A leading positive psychology expert explains that while part of happiness may be affected by outside factors, including our genetics, a substantial part of our happiness can be influenced by how we think and what we do.

Big Potential: How Transforming the Pursuit of Success Raises Our Achievement, Happiness and Well-Being – Shawn Achor
Big potential is what can be achieved by working together.

Messy: The Power of Disorder to Transform Our Lives – Tim Harford
How the human qualities we value – creativity, responsiveness, and resilience are integral to the disorder, confusion, and disarray that produce them.

Meditations – Marcus Aurelius
A Roman Emperor provides guidance for daily living. Its principles are as applicable today as they were in Roman times.

Stumbling on Happiness – Dan Gilbert
The Harvard psychologist describes the problems of foresight that cause each of us to misconceive our tomorrows and misestimate our satisfactions.

The 7 Habits of Highly Effective People – Stephen Covey
How to incorporate these critical habits into a plan for accomplishing your goals.

Little Bets: How Breakthrough Ideas Emerge from Small Discoveries – Peter Sims
The benefits of trying things in low risk tests to be guided where to go next.

Happiness: Unlocking The Mysteries of Psychological Wealth – Ed Diener and Robert Biswas-Diener
Challenges the present thinking of the causes and consequences of happiness and redefines our modern notions of it.

Your Best Life Now: 7 Steps To Living Life at Your Full Potential – Joel Osteen
The famous television evangelist provides suggestions for living a positive life. Christians will be able to easily relate to the beneficial message this book contains, *but it can benefit anyone of any faith or of none.*

A New Earth: Awakening to Your Life's Purpose – Eckhart Tolle
A step-by-step presentation to help you discover your guiding purposes. Even though this book was highly promoted by Oprah Winfrey, it would be a mistake to think that it is only a women's book. Anyone can benefit from it.

Blink – Malcolm Gladwell

Great stories emphasizing that good decisions can often be made by thin slicing, using a small amount of information that leads to a decision that might be the same as if more research were done in making it.

George Foreman's Guide to Life – George Foreman

Not just a man's book, nor is it a boxing book. It's one that can benefit anyone. Contains excellent practical advice for getting the most out of life.

Finding Meaning in the Second Half of Life: How to Finally Really Grow Up – James Hollis

Dr. Hollis offers excellent advice for making the most out of the end game.

Thinking Fast and Slow – Daniel Kahneman

An excellent and thoughtful exposition on different types of thinking and how to improve our decision making.

Portraits of Courage – George W. Bush

Provides inspiring biographies of disabled veterans, each accompanied by portraits painted by our 43rd President.

Character Is Destiny – John McCain

Provides excellent models for many positive character traits.

Other Books by Lawrence J. Danks

Finding Happiness and Success: Innovation, Motivation, Reinvention, Becoming A Better You
A guide to developing your best self through a summarized review and constructive commentary of proven principles from positive psychology and management.

Your Unfinished Life: The Classic and Timeless Guide to Finding Happiness and Success Through Kindness
Ever feel as if part of you is missing? Be the person you might never have become. There's still time left in your unfinished life. Finding happiness and achieving success, motivation, inspiration, kindness and service to others, and achieving increased fulfillment. Includes summaries of two classic works on kindness by Jean Guibert and Frederick Faber with author's commentary. Inspiring quotes from Marcus Aurelius, Mother Teresa, The Dalai Lama, George Foreman, Joel Osteen, Martin Seligman, Stephen Covey, Eckhardt Tolle, and many others. Revealing insights to lead you to your highest and most fulfilled self, so your unplayed music won't die inside you.

Finding the Right Man for You: Dating Advice for Women
Finding the Right Man for You helps women evaluate their current situation, provides support in dealing with divorce or the death of a partner, addresses fear and self-doubt, recommends what to look for in a man, provides perspectives on sex and intimacy, offers many suggestions on how to meet men, offers online dating tips and guidance in answering dating questionnaires and in writing personal statements. Recommendations on dating for women who have children and work pressures, personal and financial safety, how to guard against men who lie, health and dating, finding happiness with or without a man, finding love and romance, and

ultimately making a decision about a man. The book has been reviewed by female reviewers and advisors who have offered their valuable insights and experiences. It's motivational and supportive and provides inspiration through memorable stories and powerful quotations.

For College Students: You and Your Future
To find success and happiness in life, there are certain things college students should be doing, and not be doing, that can contribute mightily to achieving their goals. Lawrence J Danks has been a full-time and adjunct college professor for over forty years. Let his long-term experience with college students help you or your favorite college student with this self-help guide. Sample topics include:

- College selection and return on investment
- What is the best college for you?
- Finding your place in life
- Nine steps to success
- Finding a job
- Suggested career fields
- Obstacles to success
- How much money do you want to make?
- What's more important than money?

Made in the USA
Columbia, SC
12 November 2018